SWAMI KRIPALU'S
LADDER OF YOGA

SWAMI KRIPALU'S

LADDER of YOGA

RICHARD FAULDS

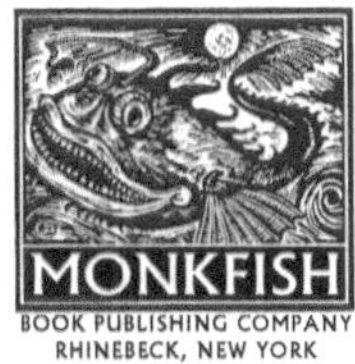

MONKFISH
BOOK PUBLISHING COMPANY
RHINEBECK, NEW YORK

The archival materials upon which this book is based are used by permission of Kripalu Center for Yoga & Health, Stockbridge, MA, kripalu.org. All the photographs of Swami Kripalu appearing in this book are used by permission. The cover shot and photos of Swami Kripalu practicing yoga postures and mudras previously appeared in *Asana and Mudra* (Red Elixir, an imprint of Monkfish Books Publishing Company, 2018). For a digital library that includes many of Swami Kripalu's original works see https://naturalmeditation.online. *Asana and Mudra* is available to purchase at Amazon.com All other photographs are from the private collection of the author unless otherwise noted in the caption. For a wealth of photographs and information about the life and teachings of Swami Kripalu visit www.swamikripalvananda.org.

Paperback ISBN 9781966608134
eBook ISBN 9781966608141

Library of Congress Cataloging-in-Publication Data Pending

Book and cover design by Colin Rolfe

Monkfish Book Publishing Company
22 East Market Street, Suite 304
Rhinebeck, New York 12572
(845) 876-4861
monkfishpublishing.com

If humankind wants to rise above the darkness of ignorance to reach the light of knowledge, there is a need for a ladder. That ladder is yoga.

–Swami Kripalu

CONTENTS

NOTE TO THE READER

This is the third volume in a trilogy of Swami Kripalu books written in the dozen years since I retired as a staff member of Kripalu Center for Yoga & Health, the largest yoga-based retreat and program center in North America. *Dharma Then Moksha: The Untold Story of Swami Kripalu* is an illustrated recounting of his remarkable life story. *Swami Kripalu's Yoga of Success and Self-Realization* presents his foundational teachings with an emphasis on the essentials of yoga philosophy and the healthy lifestyle integral to successful spiritual practice. This third volume details his guidance on *asana* (postures), *pranayama* (yogic breathing), and the meditative techniques meant to raise consciousness through a series of quantum-like steps that transform one's sense of self. Along with providing the knowledge needed to make good use of these tools, it retraces the efforts of myself and others—sometimes effectively and other times unsuccessfully—to progress along Swami Kripalu's path of yoga through the type of systematic practice he valued so highly.

Readers of these previous volumes know that Swami Kripalu was a reclusive sage renowned in his native India as a humanitarian saint who startled his many followers by coming to America in 1977. Residing at the original Kripalu Yoga Ashram in Sumneytown, Pennsylvania, he spent the final four years of his life pursuing the end stages of yoga described in the traditional texts but seldom achieved by today's practitioners. I met Swami Kripalu there in May of 1981, two days after graduating from college, an encounter that set me on the path of yoga just as I was crossing the threshold into adulthood. Swami Kripalu was long past accepting students. The only way to join his yoga lineage was to be initiated by his close disciple, Yogi Amrit Desai,[1] which my wife Danna and I did early in our relationship. Forty-five years later, we are still studying and practicing the path that Swami Kripalu modeled and taught.

The chief content of all these books is not my narrative text but the extensive body of quotations, excerpts, and teaching stories that remain as close as possible to Swami Kripalu's words. Every effort has been made to retain his distinctive voice and subtlety of expression. To convey a whole message on a particular topic, it was often necessary to combine material drawn from different sources and express them in a single narrative. Rather than academic literalness, I strove to present Swami Kripalu's guidance in a straightforward fashion true to the original.

As a reader, it's important to know that virtually all of the material depicted in *italics* is drawn from Swami Kripalu's legacy of published works, scholarly discourses, transcribed talks, and personal correspondence. This includes the epigraphs that open each chapter and the segregated sections interspersed throughout the text. I tried to moderate my use of the Sanskrit terms that permeate the original sources, italicizing and defining important ones for readers eager to learn more, while respecting those who want things said in plain English. In places where Swami Kripalu's name is repeated often, it is shortened to SK for ease of reading.

Being familiar with contemporary yogic literature, I can say this book's content is noteworthy for addressing a host of esoteric topics in a sensible manner that enables their guiding principles to be applied on the mat and cushion. Make no mistake, these are potent teachings shared by Swami Kripalu to bring the mysteries of yoga alive for his students. They are preserved and presented here to empower the practice of dedicated yogis everywhere.

[1] Yogi Amrit Desai was born in the Gujarat village of Halol, India, where he met Swami Kripalu as a boy. After emigrating to America in the 1960s to attend the Philadelphia College of Art, Desai founded a yoga ashram in Pennsylvania and named it after his teacher. The ashram later became Kripalu Center for Yoga & Health, now located in Stockbridge, Massachusetts.

AUTHOR'S PREFACE

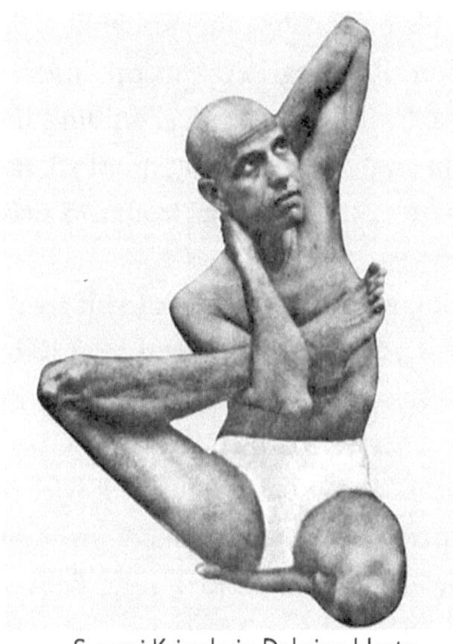

Swami Kripalu in Daksina Hasta Catuskonasana.

It's a rare soul who would not be stretched beyond their limits in treading the yogic path that Swami Kripalu walked. But that rather obvious fact did not stop me and a host of ashram residents from trying to follow in his footsteps. In falling short, many practical lessons were learned that aided in the transmission of yoga to the West. This is why a small cast of ashram characters are introduced in the pages that follow and the stories surrounding them recounted. But it was only years later, while researching this book and distilling one of SK's lectures into the following excerpt, that an alternative and better approach than emulating him occurred to me.

The ancient Indian yogis sustained themselves by asking for alms from householders. Grateful to receive material support, the yogis provided guidance so the householders could advance spiritually. Thus began a synergistic arrangement that has continued for time immemorial. The gurus of old were complete teachers able to acquaint a student with all the yogic approaches. After a student chose a particular yogic pathway, the guru would provide the specialized guidance needed to commence its practice. Then as the student moved from one stage of yoga to another, the guru would explain both the obstructions being removed and the mysteries being revealed. With their doubts resolved and the way ahead cleared of obstacles, the progress of such a student was never delayed or brought to a standstill. A householder yogi, blessed by such a teacher, could make remarkable progress.

Right on the heels of making this statement, SK was quick to lament: *But today, only incomplete teachers are available who teach from their experience of following a particular path to a preliminary point.* After all my research, I had learned enough about his personality and teaching style to not get sidetracked by this deflection. Reading between the lines, I grew certain that this excerpt gave voice to the age-old ideal guiding his efforts as a modern teacher. Gazing through this lens, my mind struggled to take in the implications of examining his teachings from this new perspective.

What if Swami Kripalu was not trying to enroll anyone into an arduous renunciate practice? What if he was providing us a broad body of instruction in which to find the stage-by-stage guidance we needed to advance along our particular and idiosyncratic paths? What if SK was neither disciplinarian nor taskmaster, but a compassionate well-wisher who only wanted to leverage the experience he had gained through his extraordinary yoga to make our ordinary householder yoga deliver remarkable results?

The more I contemplated these questions, the more confident I felt in answering each of them in the affirmative. Along with being logically consistent, it was true to my experience. Ever since meeting Swami Kripalu, I had practiced yoga drawing on many resources. But I always found myself returning to his teachings as the lantern needed to navigate my way through whatever new and unknown landscape I happened to be passing.

Now, with this book going to press, I encourage you as a reader to adopt this perspective too. Instead of struggling to understand and embody the entirety of what SK taught, be on the lookout for the gems that illumine your path in the moment. And as your practice of yoga evolves, remember that you can come back to these teachings whenever a new stage of growth is calling you to explore deeper or farther. Guided in this way, may your practice lead you rung-by-rung into the higher stages of yoga just as he said was possible: *without ever being delayed or brought to a standstill.*

RICHARD FAULDS
Greenville, Virginia

CHAPTER 1

INTRODUCING THE LADDER OF YOGA

Householders are taught the limbs of yoga one by one. This method of instruction is ancient and totally in accord with the experience of the rishis and sages. Through it a yogi living in society may travel fearlessly on the path of incremental progress. By grasping the eight limbs of yoga like the rungs of a ladder, a diligent householder can ascend this path all the way to samadhi.

Swami Kripalu encouraged the type of body-based yoga popular today as a time-tested way to remedy common illnesses and attain good health. Yet he was quick to add that the very same yoga, when practiced with an orienting view and supportive lifestyle, could do considerably more than prevent disease and boost vitality. Knowing firsthand that yoga was designed to propel a student through a progression of stages that psychology regards as a sequence of human development, SK taught yoga as a method of restoring health, catalyzing psychological growth, and stepping beyond the mind's limits into the realm of spiritual awakening. In explaining the mechanism behind yoga's elevating effect, he subscribed to its traditional model of energy anatomy, which meshed well with his own experience.

In yogic texts both ancient and modern, there are descriptions of various energy centers that lie dormant in the body. Through the science of yoga, these centers can be activated and through them their corresponding nerve plexus, glands, and organs stimulated. As each center is brought to life, a ladder is formed. Regardless of what type of yoga is practiced, a yogi's ascent of this ladder must begin at the lowest center. The great primal power coalesced there

> *must be made active and raised to successively higher centers. A yogi who enlivens the uppermost center has reached the ladder's highest rung. Nothing beyond that need be done. An aspiring student must accept the support of this ladder, as it is only through ascending it that yoga's profound benefits are produced.*

While the idea of waking up a primal power may sound exotic, its roots are decidedly down to earth. Indian culture is grounded in an agrarian mindset in which every farmer sees how certain animals from a litter, and plants in a crop of seedlings, display unusual vigor. If the needs of these hardy plants and animals are well-tended, they reliably grow into exceptional specimens. Few of us are born with such vigor, so the yogic sages experimented to see if the practice of various disciplines could jump-start the primal power of everyone. Through careful trial and error, they discovered the life force of the body can be raised to high levels of activity in a wide range of individuals. Where the growth of plants and animals reaches a natural limit at physical maturity, the nervous system development of a human being can continue over the course of a lifetime. That's what allows this *energy-based yoga* to serve as the biological basis for a potent form of spirituality.

Farmers know the maturation of animals follows a definite biological template. The sages saw that the higher growth of a human being also unfolds in accord with an organic pattern, but only if the life force is kept strong by the ongoing practice of these disciplines. On the path Swami Kripalu taught, the template that guides the process of healing, self-development, and spiritual awakening is the ladder of yoga. In order to ascend and reach to its upper rungs, a person must learn to cultivate their energetic vitality by living in cooperation with the primal energies underlying the body and mind.[1]

[1] This paragraph delineates the core of Swami Kripalu's approach to yoga, which in India is known by many names. He avoided attaching any particular label to it, believing that all authentic yoga lineages directly or indirectly utilize this same bio-psycho-spiritual mechanism. One name he used is *sahaja yoga*, which means *natural yoga*. In rare individuals like SK, the triggering of the primal force brings forth all the techniques needed to keep it active and working at progressively higher levels. These techniques are done intuitively and without any need for external instruction. For these individuals, yoga practice becomes a natural process of surrendering ever more deeply to the power and intelligence of this awakened energy. Most people, however, need to be taught these techniques as yoga students, after which they are

Having studied many versions of this model, I can say that Swami Kripalu's view of how the ladder of yoga is ascended by students he categorized as either *renunciates* or *householders* is unique. For renunciate monks and nuns practicing yoga intensively as their sole vocation in life, the awakening of the primal power is meant to be strong and sudden, unfolding from there in a similar manner to what SK experienced as a swami and detailed in his biography.[2] For those practicing yoga in the midst of a career and family life, a gradual activation is considered much more desirable. SK often said that a householder's movement up the ladder of yoga can be so slow and steady that they may not sense anything unusual is happening, yet the signs of this activation will eventually become evident in all areas of their life.

The ancient sages scaled this ladder of yoga to its highest rung and understood it thoroughly. They were able to provide the necessary instruction to make all their students pilgrims on the path of yoga, but the forest dwellers (renunciates) and town-dwellers (householders) were placed in different study groups. Householders were taught the limbs of yoga one-by-one to activate the primal power in its partial and tolerable form. They knew well that this was the correct way for students living a life in society to progress spiritually. To presume these sages were acting improperly is to make a mistake. A householder performing their daily yoga routine may doubt that anything is happening. As a result, they may lose inspiration before the truth of their changing inner condition becomes discernible. A partial activation of the primal power will eventually be reflected in the emergence of extraordinary capacities and qualities, but only if practice is continued into yoga's upper rungs.

---

encouraged to feel their way into the volitional application of them that best meets their unique and evolving needs. One traditional name for this approach is *kundalini yoga*, however that term is used by numerous yoga schools in the West to describe divergent styles. Prominent among them is the yoga of the Sikh religious tradition brought to America by Yogi Bhajan, which uses the brand name Kundalini Yoga to promote its system of movements, breathing exercises, and mantra chanting. Although SK was clearly teaching a traditional form of kundalini yoga, that term is not used in this book to avoid confusion.

[2] For more on the energy awakening that Swami Kripalu experienced, see *Dharma Then Moksha*, Chapters 4 and 5.

Encountering this teaching, I asked myself an obvious question, "What exactly is an ordinary spiritual seeker like me to do?" Eventually, I learned the answer is simple. Continue doing your yoga, mindfully performing the basic techniques in the framework of a supportive lifestyle, and trust the power of the practices to do their inner work.

This ladder was not created by the yogis. Each soul descends it to take birth and will ascend it again at death. Discovering it inside themselves, great yogis scaled it to realization and liberation. All you as a householder student need to know is that this ladder exists within you. A ladder doesn't have one step—it has many steps—so do not imagine that wherever you happen to be on this ladder is the end. Perform your everyday routine of spiritual practices while keenly observing your mind, and your awareness will steadily grow more penetrating. This way the subtler aspects of the basic techniques will become clear to you. Applying this knowledge in practice, the next rung of the ladder will come into reach. It is only through the diligent practice of yoga's elemental techniques that its advanced techniques are generated.

The next few chapters present Swami Kripalu's teachings on a topic he called *yogic anatomy*. Later chapters track the progression of techniques prescribed by the sages to activate the primal force, enliven the energy centers, and ascend the ladder of yoga. While scaling a ladder sounds like hard work, SK made sure his students knew that there is always an element of effortlessness and grace involved.

When I landed in New York, I saw my first escalator. Looking at it, I understood immediately that this was a ladder that a person doesn't have to climb. Its machinery is designed to take you up. So I got on the first step and just stood. As it started moving upward, I thought to myself, "This is the cleverness of man." Don't you think God would also have this same intelligence? The experience that a person is climbing the ladder of yoga is only an illusion. Simply take the first step and allow the escalating to be done by the science of yoga.

CHAPTER 2

THE YOGIC BODY

Everyone knows how medical researchers developed the science of anatomy through the dissection of dead bodies. In a similar way, the yogis developed a science of subtle energy by exploring their living bodies. Given their differing methods, it is natural that each of these systems has its own viewpoint. Even so, a general understanding is reflected in these two approaches that every yogic aspirant should possess.

A few years into our residency, all the ashram's yoga teachers gathered in the main chapel for a special session. After some warm-ups and vigorous breathing exercises, we were guided through a series of seven yoga postures. Each pose was held for several minutes, during which we chanted a one syllable "seed mantra" and visualized energy streaming to the area of the body it effected. We were told the physical stimulation of the posture, sound vibration of the mantra, and targeted mental focus would awaken our chakras.

Spurred on by this promise, everyone pulled out the stops. This made for a cathartic session, but thinking back I have to chuckle. It's not the techniques that were lacking. It's that we didn't possess the understanding required to use them wisely. While all the knowledge we needed was right there in Swami Kripalu's teachings, immaturity led us to pursue fantastical notions over the real potential of an informed yoga practice. While none of us turned into light beings that day, the story of our failed efforts may help you engage the topic of yogic anatomy with a little more discernment than we were able to muster.

The chakra model was originally a closely guarded yogic secret made known only to initiates. Nowadays the notion that our physical body is undergirded by an energy body marked by a constellation of spiraling energy centers is commonplace. But what does it really signify? And how can it be usefully applied? SK answered these questions quite directly. But as I began to understand the implications of what he was saying, two overriding questions formed in my mind. Where exactly did his knowledge come from? And how trustworthy was it?

MERGING YOGIC EXPERIENCE AND MODERN SCIENCE

I knew that Swami Kripalu had spent years studying yoga's authoritative texts, which describe the *yogic body* through a rich mix of symbols and metaphors created to guide practice and explain its energetic effects. Yet this alone did not account for the full scope of his teachings. It was clear that a portion of his knowledge of the *nadis* (energy channels), *chakras* (energy centers), and *granthis* (constricting knots) was direct and experiential. In this excerpt, he describes the activation process in traditional terms, while also including elements from his first-person practice.

According to the science of yoga, there are 72,000 energy channels and numerous chakras. But it is difficult to accept this science until the presence of these subtle channels and centers is revealed in the meditative state. The consciousness of an adept yogi is able to wander freely through this vast internal network. This ability comes through the practice of postures, pranayama, and moderate diet, which causes the impurities that block these channels to dwindle. As the channels open, the piercing of the three granthis begins and proceeds upward from the belly to the brow. As this movement gains strength, the chakras start to develop, that is they blossom into greater activity. But a few months of practice is not enough for this to occur. The scriptures say that a minimum of twelve years is required. Success in a task like this is best regarded as dependent on grace and not the result of hard labor. So I pray daily to my nadis, chakras, and granthis, saying "I can only traverse the path of yoga with your help. Please have mercy on me and reveal your secrets."

In some places, the introspective knowledge that Swami Kripalu appears to have received strained my limits of credulity. Here is one of many examples.

Once I was watching my blood flow through my blood vessels when I heard a voice say, "I am your lymph," and noticed right away how it was colorless and oozing out of the capillaries. The lymphatic vessels carried me inside them, and I experienced how the small capillaries flow into larger and larger passageways that empty into two large ducts, where the lymph again mixes with the blood. Traveling through the lymphatic vessels, I encountered many lymph glands and saw how the white blood cells have a right of way that enables them to enter one end and leave through another. Each gland is full of these cells, which allows them to destroy germs and prevent disease. This how the lymph introduced itself to me.

At first, I wasn't sure what to make of these statements. Especially when SK blended his yogic experiences with information gleaned from his study of Western anatomy and physiology.[1] The amount of biological information packed into these textbook-like accounts made me doubt their authenticity. Eventually I came to understand that he was coupling meditative introspection with techniques like visualization and inner-dialoguing to enhance his self-exploration. Afterward, he drew on the terminology of the health sciences to help convey his experiences. This reflects the overall approach he recommended of using yogic tools to subjectively investigate the subtle body, while also learning from objective perspectives. In this excerpt, he tries to bridge these worlds.

The knowledge of the energy centers arose in ancient times. At present, their study can be made on the basis of science. Physiology recognizes the different systems of the body. We may say that the first chakra is the excretory system. The second is the reproductive system. The third is the digestive system. The fourth is the respiratory and circulatory systems. The sixth and seventh chakras are different aspects of the brain and nervous system. Taken together, the seven chakras comprise the endocrine system, all of which are upheld by the skeletal and muscular systems. From the viewpoint of yoga, the flow of life energy through the various channels and centers is

[1] This is most evident in his encyclopedic work, *Asana and Mudra.*

most important. From the viewpoint of physiology and kinesiology, the function of the nerve plexuses, glands, muscles, and joints is most important. But yoga involves more than the study of the physical body and health. It includes knowledge of the mind, the soul, and the nature of the universe. All of this knowledge constitutes the spiritual science of yoga, which was gained by the exploration of the living body, mind, and consciousness. Today East and West are getting to know each other, and a student well-versed in yoga can practice its techniques while also taking into consideration the discoveries of modern science.

The above excerpts demonstrate how Swami Kripalu braided three strands into his teaching of energy anatomy: the traditional yogic model, his subjective inner experience, and Western science. The next two chapters draw heavily on those teachings to present an energetic template for yoga practice that is grounded in time-tested symbolism but integrates useful scientific knowledge.

THE SUBTLE BODY

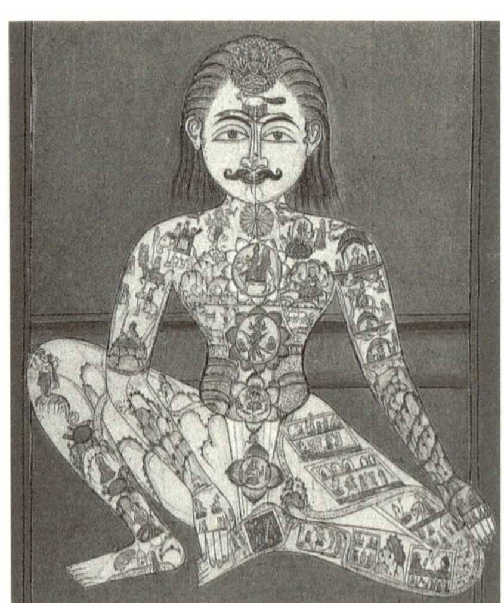

A visual depiction of the subtle body from an 1899 Yoga manuscript called the Jogapradipika. Source: Wiki Commons.

While the chakras tend to get all the attention, they are one component of a larger whole called the *subtle body* (*sukshma sharira*). Most of us have seen the detailed maps of the meridians depicted by the Chinese sages who developed acupuncture. The Indian sages charted the internal flow of life energies in a similar fashion and considered the subtle body the intermediary link through which the soul vitalizes the material body. They believed the current state of a person's subtle body is reflected in their health, behavior patterns, and favored modes of being. But the yogis emphasized a positive teaching: the enlivened subtle body that results from focused yoga practice can serve as a matrix for higher consciousness, better health, and improved functioning.

The yogic texts describe a human being as having multiple bodies, but the two basic categories of gross (sthula) and subtle (sukshma) are inclusive of all. The gross aspect of a human being is the outer physical body, which internally includes many blood vessels, nerve pathways, nerve plexuses, and organs. The subtle aspect is the prana body (body of life energy), which includes the nadis (tubes) and chakras (wheels). The subtlest aspect of a human being is the mental body (antahkarana), which includes the full spectrum of ordinary and extraordinary mind states. All of these bodies derive their power from the immaterial soul (atman) and can be made more dynamic through yogic techniques. Adept yogis consider knowledge of the subtle body to be better than that of the gross body, because this knowledge can be applied in postures and pranayama to make the life force very strong. In the same way, they consider knowledge of the mental body to be superior to that of the subtle body, because by applying it in meditation a revelatory state of one-pointed consciousness can be brought about. One who understands this sees that the subtle body plays an essential intermediary role in the process of yoga. Practice begins in the gross body, then shifts into the subtle body, and eventually enters the domain of mind to access the soul.

Yoga operates on the premise that the subtle body is malleable and can be shaped by a combination of conscious breathing, bodily position, attention, and intention. This idea meshes with current notions of neuroplasticity and neurogenesis.[2] Working with a clear template of how energy is meant to flow through the system makes it easier to engage the mind in focused asana and pranayama practice. Later on, it informs and empowers techniques including visualization and meditation. The heightened inner flow of life energy that results from these practices is

[2] Neuroplasticity is an umbrella term referring to the brain's ongoing ability to change, adapt, and reorganize synaptic connections in response to experience. Neurogenesis is the formation of entirely new neurons and neural pathways in the adult brain, which until recently was thought impossible.

the invisible engine of the transformative process, catalyzing the physical, emotional, and mental effects that differentiate yoga from mechanically-done calisthenics and other forms of exercise as ordinarily practiced.

THREE PRINCIPAL PATHWAYS

The basic component of the subtle body is an intricate network of nadis or energy pathways that branch off into ever-smaller channels, much like the circulatory system. The prevailing yogic model describes three principal pathways, fourteen major branches, 72,000 secondary channels, and 350,000 minute conduits. Swami Kripalu spoke of the nadis broadly as a *complex of tubes* that includes all the nerves and interior bodily passages through which proprioceptive awareness can flow.[3] The sheer number of these pathways reflects yoga's affirmation of our incredible capacity for self-awareness when the flow of energy through the subtle body is unobstructed. As we inhale through the nostrils to take in oxygen and fuel the metabolism of the physical body, yoga teaches that we also absorb prana to sustain the dynamic aliveness of the subtle body.

The number of energy channels is legion but only three nadis figure prominently in the practice of yoga. The solar or heating channel is on the right side. The lunar or cooling channel is on the left side. Between these two dwells the central channel, which in most bodies is blocked by an accumulation of physical, emotional, and mental impurities. This leaves only the right and left channels active. Through the practice of postures and pranayama, life energy is made to flow through the heating and cooling channels more easily. As a result, all the 72,000 nadis begin to purify. Health improves and the flow of energy through the complex of peripheral channels grows regular and equalized. Only after this is accomplished

[3] The Latin word *propius* means "one's own." Proprioception is the medical term for the innate ability of individuals to sense the stimuli produced within their own organism, especially those connected with the position and movement of the body. Yoga offers a greatly expanded version of this idea. The term *nadi* appears in the Katha Upanishad, which describes it as a perceptible flow of sensation. Centuries later in the hatha yoga texts, the emphasis shifts to seeing nadis as tubes in the effort to map the anatomy of the subtle body. Depth practice is best supported by the original definition.

does the dark condition of the mind fade away and its capacity to become stable and one-pointed arise.

THE THREE PRICNIPAL PATHWAYS

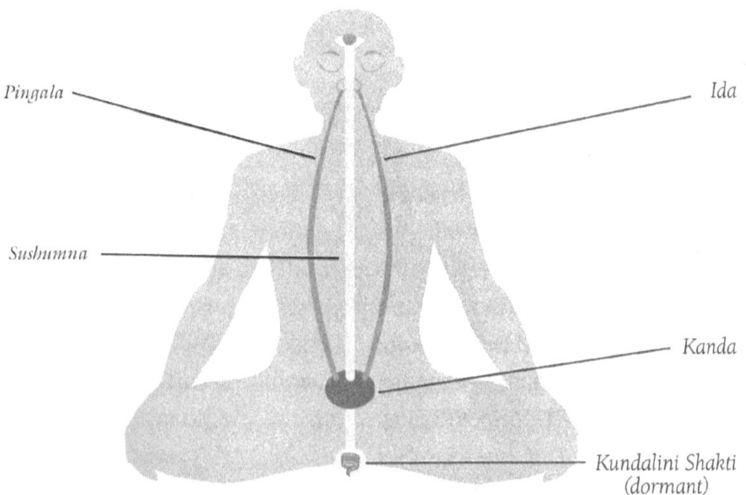

The three principal pathways of the subtle body as depicted by SK with a dormant Kundalini Shakti. Source: *Kripalu Yoga: A Guide to Practice On and Off the Mat* (Bantam Books 2005, 233.)

The *pingala nadi* (solar or heating channel) is on the right side. The *ida nadi* (lunar or cooling channel) is on the left side. Swami Kripalu described these two major peripheral channels as distinct energy-flows running vertically and parallel to the spine. His visual depictions show them connecting the nostrils to the kanda, a word meaning "bulb," which is the egg-shaped origin point of all the energy pathways located slightly below the navel. Other yoga schools depict these channels as intimately-related energies crisscrossing the spine and ending at the "third eye" or point between the eyebrows.

Yoga's power to shift consciousness appears to stem from its ability to use the heating and cooling channels to alter the function of the nervous system. Neurologically, the heating pathway is thought to correspond to the sympathetic branch of the autonomic nervous system, which is responsible for narrowing the focus of attention and arousing the body to action. The cooling pathway is thought to correspond to its parasympathetic branch, which widens the aperture of awareness, calms the body, and enables us to relax, digest, and heal. When vital energy flows smoothly and evenly through these two pathways, the mind is balanced, attentive, and free of agitation. Although a rarity in our distracted world, yoga considers this our normal state of healthy functioning.

Body-based yoga techniques to foster this state of inner balance include rocking, twisting, and scissoring movements that repeatedly stimulate one side of the body and then the other. Cross-crawl movements that move opposite arms and legs in ways that cross over the midline of the body are another type of integrating movement pattern known by science to improve cognitive function. There is a catch-all name for these body-based balancing techniques: bilateral stimulation. But by far the most direct and effective yogic method of working with the two sides of the nervous system is breath-based pranayama as explained in later chapters and appendixes.

The central channel or *sushumna nadi* is the subtle body's chief pathway running from the perineum to the crown of the head through the interior of the spinal column.[4] It's noteworthy that all schools of yoga describe this nadi as being blocked in most people. When these blocks are cleared and energy is made to flow along or through the central channel, the activity of the two peripheral pathways is greatly diminished. As the mind and nervous system grow quiet, inner awareness is heightened, which enables meditation to become highly focused. This is the mechanism underlying the experience of introversion, which makes a spectrum of meditative states and eventually non-dual awareness accessible.

The most common technique to encourage energy to flow through the central channel is directing attention to the spot between the eyebrows, or visualizing energy flowing from root to crown, both of which are often done in combination with specific breathing exercises. Swami Kripalu explained how this can also be accomplished by the skillful use of postures, a teaching I've never seen elsewhere.

Many yoga asanas are practiced on two sides by alternating the position of the torso and limbs. This places pressure first on one side

[4] The yogis describe the spinal column as having a hollow core. While anatomically incorrect, this idea might reflect the fact that nerves cannot feel themselves. The interior of the spine could have occurred to the yogis as an introspective void until a sensation of energy flowing through it was generated by visualization and other yogic techniques.

of the body, and then on the other. Whenever the left side is pressed, the life force is made to move strongly through the right channel. All its associated functions become more active as the left channel is momentarily suppressed. In the same way, when the right side is pressed, the life force is made to move strongly through the left channel. All its associated functions become more active as the right channel is momentarily suppressed. In other asanas, both sides are pressed simultaneously. If these both-side poses are done intensively and held, the life force will stop flowing in both the right and left channels. This is one way it can be made to begin to flow through the central channel, which has a steadying effect on the mind.

It's common for yoga instructors to pause a class after a two-sided posture has been performed on one side and ask students to notice if that side of the body feels different than the other. After both sides are done, attention might be directed to the mid-line of the body. The purpose of this exercise is to develop the proprioceptive ability to sense the relative degree of openness in the two halves of the gross and subtle bodies, while also suggesting the potential for a mid-line awakening.

ENERGY BLOCKS

Yoga teaches that the life energy continually moving through the subtle body is often constricted by three nerve tangles in the belly, throat, and head. These are the *granthis*, a word meaning knot. A granthi can be likened to the ball of hair and dirt that clogs a bathroom drain. Energy can also be blocked by localized obstructions at vital points called *marmans*. Together these knots slow the flow of life force moving through the inner pathways to a trickle, dulling the vitality of physical tissues and causing a buildup of waste products.[5] From the vantage point of the subtle body, a primary purpose of yoga practice is to untangle these regional knots and remove any localized obstructions to free up the flow of life force through the system. The cleansing process and revitalization of the body-mind it engenders is called *shuddhi* or purification.

[5] Some yogic texts say the granthis are spots where the soul is tied to the material body. This curious idea may have arisen to explain how untying these knots can quickly bring a liberating experience of spiritual awakening.

Yoga science describes three granthis or knots that an aspirant must untie to realize the Self. The ancient yogis attributed great importance to these granthis, as they believed that all the nadis of the subtle body are controlled by them. Today we could say that a granthi is a complex of nerves whose degree of function is reflected in our predominant state of consciousness, whether lethargic, active, or serene. The first knot is in the region of the lower chakras. It is physically centered in the genitals, where procreation takes place, and controls the reproductive and excretory systems. The second knot is in the region of the throat chakra. Physically it is centered in the mouth, tongue, and sublingual glands, through which the body receives sustenance. Whenever we take food, it is this granthi that is operating. The third knot is in the region of the brow chakra. Physically it is centered in the forebrain, through which we exercise our will to act. When the unconscious power of these granthis is dominant, the conscious mind is rendered feeble and a person feels helplessly drawn by the instinctual forces of nature to engage in all sorts of habitual and harmful actions. When an aspirant becomes aware of these knots and works to untie them, they gain a greater degree of autonomy and the power to control the senses. This enables them to bring these formerly unconscious forces of nature expressing through the granthis into balance and use them consciously to evolve.

Purification is a consistent theme in Swami Kripalu's yoga, and one that must be interpreted correctly before those teachings can be properly applied. Traditional yoga says surprisingly little about what psychologists would call growth. Instead, yoga focuses on techniques that cleanse the body-mind in accord with the belief that growth will unfold naturally once the impurities have been removed and the free flow of life energy restored. What exactly are these impurities? Impurity is often taken religiously to mean sin, as in a stain or lingering effect of morally bad actions. But yogic impurities are anything and everything that blocks the free flow of life force, fosters energetic stagnation, and limits the vitality of the gross, subtle, or causal bodies. This includes a wide range of physical imbalances, emotional issues, and psychological conditions. For more on this, see the sidebar on page 90.

Utilizing this broad definition of impurity, yoga's prescription to cleanse the system is straightforward. Physical impurities are removed by regular exercise and right diet. Energetic blocks are released by a combination of asana, pranayama, and visualization. Problematic emotional and mental patterns are remedied by meditation and the self-reflection its practice entails. Viewed in this context, the three granthis reflect a level of human development that is habit-based and oriented to survival, self-protection, and satiating the senses. The granthis aren't evil, but the unconscious mode in which they operate encourages a lifestyle of indulgence that inevitably dulls vitality, suppresses growth, and undermines our long-term happiness.

Yoga teaches that all the impurities blocking the subtle channels and energy centers came about by actions generated by the granthis misusing the organs associated with them. In the same way, all the channels and centers can be purified by untangling these knots and using the organs properly. The practice of asana, and pranayama activates the life force, which starts to speedily purify the channels. Soon the process of untying the first two knots and revitalizing their associated nerve plexuses begins. Yoga shows us that most of our bodily ills are the results of bad habits and lack of self-discipline. As we correct these mistakes, our willpower gains strength. The process builds momentum and moves to the brow chakra. Untying this knot, our capacity to discern desirable from undesirable actions grows. We become free to pursue a new direction in life. If we continue to practice pranayama and meditation, we will become sensitive to the various chakras and nadis operating in the body, and the process of spiritual growth will begin.

AN EXPERIENCE OF THE GRANTHIS

After finishing my second year of law school in 1983, I was fed up with school work. Boarding a bus to Bend Oregon, I set out to bicycle a thousand miles of back roads and blue highways to my older brother's house outside of Los Angeles. Limited to what I could carry in my bike panniers, I took only the essentials. My sole luxury was a slim paperback of Swami Kripalu's teachings on energy anatomy.[6]

It felt euphoric to be unchained from my desk. On day one, I expressed my exuberance by getting up early and hightailing it out of town. After lunch, I made the strenuous seventeen mile climb up to Crater Lake then down the other side and into northern California. Within a week, I'd established a routine. Waking up, I'd visit the bathroom and return to my tiny pup tent for pranayama and meditation. Then I'd crawl out of my cozy sleeping bag to do a little standing yoga and watch the sun rise. After breakfast, I'd break camp and head out, pedaling a hundred or more miles and sleeping wherever I chose to pitch my tent.

After a week or two in the Northern California woods, I saw a flyer at a health food store for a Grateful Dead show in Valencia. Amazingly, I was able to get myself there in time to score a ticket and stash my bike. Entering the arena, I felt instantly at home with the tie-dyed multitude gathering for a night of music on the beach. As soon as the show started, I found my way to an open space populated by a free-form group of solitary dancers. The music was mesmerizing, and after an hour of vigorous movement a strange sensation arose in me and steadily grew stronger. It felt as if a sizeable tree root had come alive in my lower body. Its head was right in my crotch, with tendrils spreading down my legs. I had never moved with such a low center of gravity and enjoyed an animal-like freedom. Even as I kept dancing, I wondered what this tree root was. It felt primitive, an instinctual inner being of some kind, and one entirely oblivious of the mind-based me.

I could tell this primal being had its own wants and needs. It wasn't malevolent, just self-absorbed in an amoral way that was absolutely comfortable acting to get what it wanted, even if that meant overriding my mind and all its thoughts about right, wrong, and proper decorum. I could see that it was entirely unintegrated with my socialized personality. We were two entities living in one body. Where I had mental awareness, it had the lodestone of my life force. As I danced through the night, it took restraint for my energy not to get blatantly sexual as there was a strong pull in that direction. To counter it, I closed my eyes and kept this "root

[6] The book was *Krpalupanisad*, which I read several times during the trip, a likely factor in generating the experience of the granthis that ensued.

being" occupied by moving with more and more abandon. When the show ended, I walked out of the arena feeling remarkably alive and was relieved to find my bicycle and possessions undisturbed. Within an hour, the salt air had put me into a sound sleep. I woke the next morning to find myself back to normal. The root being had gone underground again.

All these years later, I see this as my inaugural encounter with the impulsive consciousness of the first granthi. I don't think my steady householder practice has done much to aggressively "pierce the knots" in the way that hatha yoga suggests is possible, but it has made me a more integrated person able to express the instinctual energies of the granthis from a higher level of development.

BE A DISCERNING STUDENT

With brain researchers using EKGs and FMRIs to shed objective light on how yoga works, a contemporary student might wonder if Swami Kripalu's age-old yogic teachings are still relevant. After all, doesn't his adoption of a scientific mindset imply that the nadis and chakras are outdated depictions of the nervous and endocrine systems? Even if we accept this modern definition as correct, it is important to remember that yoga practice is meant to rewire the body-mind, reconfigure its network of neural pathways, alter the hormone secretion of endocrine glands, and awaken dormant brain centers, all to catalyze specific shifts in consciousness. The traditional model describes how it feels to work directly with the body's energetic circuitry to accomplish these tasks.

Anyone who has viewed an MRI video showing a person's nervous system lighting up in response to contemplative practice will conclude that these pioneering yogis were on to something. In my experience, the models they developed should not be abandoned lightly. Swami Kripalu respected Western science for its many discoveries. But he also believed that material science has its limits.

Today the gross side of yoga is freely available to the public. This is appropriate for most practitioners, as their concerns are confined to physical fitness. Yet there are a sizeable number of individuals with greater capability who can benefit from yoga's subtle side. Yogic texts clearly distinguish the gross body from the subtle body and its energy centers. But how can this subtle knowledge be conveyed to people versed only in material science? I have asked myself this question because only under the influence of the subtle body does a practitioner become luminous. Only this subtle yoga causes the divine light to shine in the eyes, and awareness of one's real nature to dawn.

A student who closely compares the models of the subtle body utilized by today's yoga schools will find their depictions rife with contradictions. As noted earlier, SK braided together three strands in his yogic anatomy: the teachings presented in the traditional texts, his experience practicing those teachings, and the discoveries of Western science. His senior students followed suit, each adopting slight variants of SK's model that complemented their subjective experience as practitioners. Any living lineage is bound to display these kinds of differing interpretations. And it is hardly a new phenomenon. Scholars know the authors of the ancient texts disagreed on all sorts of fundamental matters, including the number of chakras. When later texts attributed a pantheon of presiding gods and goddesses, propitiating mantras, geometric shapes, and colors to the chakras to aid in yogic rituals and visualization exercises, they greatly compounded the problem.

Minor inconsistencies should not be taken to mean that any particular model is wrong. Instead, it should encourage exploration by showing that all these portrayals of yogic anatomy describe an inherently subjective experience with a range of valid interpretations. While less than perfect, remember the purpose of all these models is to provide a solid starting place for your personal introspection.

APPLYING THIS CHAPTER IN PRACTICE

Psychology has grown increasingly aware of the important role played by a person's "body image," a term used to describe the subjective mental picture and felt sense of one's own body.[7] Gazing in a full-length mirror,

[7] The term body-image was coined in 1935 by Paul Schilder, an Austrian neurologist and psychoanalyst. It is now employed across the disciplines of medicine, neuroscience, psychology, philosophy, cultural studies, and feminist studies with minor variations in use.

most of us presume that we see ourselves clearly. Yet psychologists have learned that our body image is prone to all sorts of distortions. A person of average height may experience themself as decidedly short in stature. A relatively attractive person may see themself as ugly or sexually repugnant. This phenomenon is painfully evident in a spectrum of eating disorders, including anorexia nervosa, which can lead even a dangerously thin person to see themselves as unacceptably overweight.

Psychologists define body image as a mental construct that arises from all our thoughts, feelings, and memories regarding our body as well as the cultural norms to which we are exposed. There is no direct link between it and the body of subtle energy described in yoga's traditional texts. But if we broaden our conception of the yogic body to include how the physical body feels in response to our conceptions, we can begin to understand how all sorts of contemporary people have used yoga to restore their positive body image. If we make another leap and link how the body feels with the way energy in the form of neural signals and proprioceptive awareness move through it, which is based in part upon the complex of past and present thoughts about ourselves held in the mind, we can see how yoga could be a powerful adjunct to psychotherapy.

This broader view of the subtle body is not contrary to the yoga practiced by the Indian sages. Traditional yoga included various rituals employed to purge the body-mind of guilt, shame, and feelings of unworthiness. Swami Kripalu was clearly aware of this connection between yoga, body image, and overall mental health:

Our eyes can see everything in the world clearly except ourselves. For that task, one has to use the mirror of the mind, and that mirror is often distorted. Psychology is a modern science, but the human mind has existed for millennia. People in the past knew that many physical and emotional conditions which cause grievous suffering are connected to distortions of self-seeing in the mind. Yoga included treatments that today would be considered psychology, and the use of these by yogis was well-established. Even today, the recitation of prayers and positive affirmations while performing asanas (yoga postures) can bring about a wonderful change in the way we experience our bodies and minds.

In Patanjali's classical yoga, the process of purifying and revitalizing the subtle body begins with the precepts of *yama* and *niyama*, practiced not as moral rules but as *energetic alignments* with the ethical principles the Indian sages saw as inherent in the cosmos. Its exploration continues in the subsequent limbs of *asana*, *pranayama*, *pratyahara*, *dharana*, and *dhyana*. Various forms of pranayama amplify the flow of prana through the nadis, making the reality of subtle energy easier to sense. Patterns of slow and rhythmic breathing generate pratyahara, the state of inner absorption needed for introspection to be effectively practiced. Pranayama and pratyahara make possible the practice of dharana and dhyana, in which the concentrated mind directs energy to coalesce in and move through the knots and centers. It's this progression of techniques that reliably brings the theory of the yogic body alive.

In today's posture-based yoga, the practice of asana often leads directly into sitting meditation. While a bit of conscious breathing may be done beforehand to calm the mind, the intermediate step of enlivening the subtle body through focused pranayama and pratyahara is largely skipped over. While this modern approach can produce positive results, it is a departure from the established yogic tradition as well as Swami Kripalu's teachings. That's why each limb of yoga and its full repertoire of techniques are addressed in the chapters that follow.

Although not easily explained, this process of untying the knots described by the yogis is not imaginary. A real understanding of it can be gained by inner-directed practice. If researchers were to carefully study today's adept practitioners, they might find out scientifically why the ancient yogis were absolutely correct.

CHAPTER 3

THE ENERGY CENTERS

While present in a dormant form in everyone, the existence of the chakras only becomes apparent after they are awakened to activity by yogic techniques.

The yogic conception of an inner body in which vital airs circulate through a system of channels when freed of constricting knots is truly ancient and referenced in the Vedas. Also of great antiquity is the notion that the system includes important nexus points or centers as evidenced in the early Upanishads. But the idea of an ascending set of *chakras* (wheels) or *padmas* (lotus flowers) situated along the spinal column and the subtle body's central axis is considerably more recent. It arose several centuries into the Common Era and gradually took shape in the interplay of rival Hindu and Buddhist sects during the development of what came to be known as Tantra.

The texts written by these early Tantric yogis show that opposing sects propounded a host of competing models. The simplest were one-chakra systems in which the navel or heart was the hub of a spoked wheel constrained by a single knot. But there were also three, four, nine, and eleven-chakra versions. All proved precursors to a six-chakra model that became ubiquitous around the tenth century. A historian might say the seventh or crown chakra was an exclamation point at the end of a very long sentence. It was included in the synthesis adopted by Hatha Yogis near the start of the modern era and has since been adopted by most yoga schools.[1]

[1] Clarity on the development of the yogic body remains a work in process with scholars reporting a "bewildering array of textual descriptions." See *Roots of Yoga* page 172. Tantric Hatha Yoga is a specific school of yoga based on a view of yogic anatomy attributed to the tenth-century sage Matsyendra and his chief disciple Goraksha. While some tantric techniques trace back to the first century, the texts propound-

By and large, Swami Kripalu embraced this generally-accepted model. In addition to seven primary chakras, he described two subsidiary chakras, one at the palate (*talu* chakra) and the second in the midbrain (*vyoma* or *nirvana* chakra). He also recognized vital centers in the armpits, hands, and feet.

A focus of energy channels is called a chakra. There are six bodily chakras situated along the central channel from the bottom of the spine near the anus to the mid-point between the eyebrows. Above these is a seventh chakra which cannot rightly be called bodily. Some assert there are nine chakras and that is also true, as subsidiary centers exist at the palate and in the core of the cranial cavity. A chakra can be thought of as a circular boundary that circumscribes a particular region of the body. The yogic texts correctly state that the energy centers are in the subtle body. But they can also be thought of as situated in the spinal column, with a spherical domain extending to the front of the body. For example, the navel chakra is located in the back of the body but its domain spreads forward to the digestive organs. There is a similar spreading out of all the other chakras.

While fascinating in theory, the chakra model has a functional purpose. It provides a set of what Swami Kripalu called *adharas* – bodily points on which to fixate attention during practice. It's the adharas that enable a yogi to raise their energy in a quantum series of ladder-like steps. This is the blueprint for practicing many of the asana, pranayama, and meditation techniques that he taught:

The great yogi Gorakash has pointed out nine spots for meditation: the anus, genitals, navel, heart, throat, tongue, uvula, frontal

---

ing this new conception of yogic anatomy were written between the eleventh and thirteenth centuries with some important ones composed as late as the eighteenth century. The Chinese sages who developed Daoism described three "dantians," a term that means "field of vital energy." The first is located in the belly, the second in the chest, and the third in the head. While it is generally not a good idea to cross culturally mix and match elements from different spiritual systems, this simple model is compatible with ones used by early yogis and easier for beginners to put effectively into practice.

region of the brain, and crown of the head. This was the staircase he ascended. For him, meditating meant fixing the attention in those centers and nerve plexuses while also worshipping their presiding deities. For example, Ganesh (the elephant god) is said to reside in the anal region and many symbols of him are included in the chakra situated there. To begin in meditation, one has to fix attention on the gross form of the bodily spot. In the middle-stage, the focus shifts to the subtle symbol and the energies they represent. In the end, when all the plexuses and chakras are fully active and working as one, a beyond-mind yogi does not require any gross or subtle forms (adharas) to meditate.

Adhara practice is meant to commence after a modicum of control has been wrestled away from the granthis, which reflect the powerful homeostatic force of our unconscious habits. This preliminary work is done through coupling yogic lifestyle with consistent asana, pranayama, and self-reflection. Aspirants who have readied themselves through the basic forms of these practices can use next-level versions of the same techniques that utilize the bodily points to activate one chakra, then rise above it to the next, until the chakra system is functioning as an integrated whole. SK's detailed description of this process he called *piercing the chakras* includes all the instructions needed to practice it.

THE CHAKRA SYSTEM

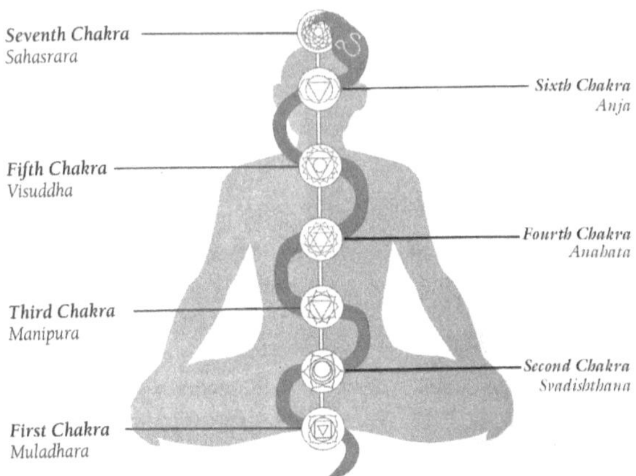

The three principal pathways of the subtle body as depicted by SK with an awakened Kundalini Shakti. Source: *Kripalu Yoga: A Guide to Practice On and Off the Mat* (Bantam Books 2005, 234).

After practicing pranayama for fifteen minutes to achieve concentration, sit in meditation pose with the palms facing up. Establish your attention on the muladhara (root) chakra and make this affirmation: "I am tapping my reservoir of primal power and transmuting its gross energies into light." This dharana (concentrated statement) is not just imagination—it will become true. Sitting upright and firm, the prana (life energy) will become steady and pierce into that part of the body (the root chakra) to start its upward course. As the prana becomes uptending, the mind will grow steady and sharp.

Stay concentrated as prana begins to rise up like water gushing from a spring and continue to affirm: "I travel upward from the root chakra to the svadhisthana (genital) chakra, then to the manipura (navel) chakra. Fix your inner gaze on your navel and watch as all weakness leaves the body. Taking its place is a sense of buoyancy and self-confidence. Continue on to the anahata (heart) chakra." Established in this chakra, what do you see? Watch as the all your peripheral energies stream through the surrounding nadis to enter the heart space and mix with the ascending prana. Notice how your respiration has naturally become slow and smooth, making the inner gaze even steadier. Center yourself there.

The clarity with which he charts the movement of the life energy gathered from the lower chakras, and now coalesced at the heart center, into the head and higher chakras is truly unusual:

Now fix the gaze on the tip of your nose, touch the tongue to the palate, and affirm as follows: "My upper chakras are being pierced by means of dharana and pranayama." Then watch as prana rises like an arrow to the visuddha (throat) and ajna (brow) chakras. Now these three centers (heart, throat, brow) are functioning as one and separate in name only.

Enter into the vyoma (space) chakra, which the yogis say is a dark cave in the center of the skull cavity. It is only from this place that the center-of-the-eyebrows meditation can begin. Once there, notice how your attention shifts to the forehead of its own accord because the prana wants to continue its ascent. Fix your gaze on the ajna (brow) chakra so the prana can establish itself in this command center of the mind.

Finally, turn your gaze up to what the yogis call the dome-of-the-sky to enter the thousand-petaled sahasra (crown) chakra. The prana may not remain steady with awareness directed above the eyebrows, but it can definitely go there. For a moment, let all the doubts and misgivings of the mind disappear. At first this experience does not last long, because the prana will soon descend, but gradually you can increase the duration of your beyond-mind meditation practice.

It is only after the piercing of the six bodily chakras that life force starts flowing freely in the central channel and the in-depth practice of yogic meditation can begin. All the impurities of the body and mind can be burned to ashes by the heat of this technique. Ascending the ladder of the chakras, one approaches the precincts of God and need not go anywhere else in search of illuminating knowledge.

AN EXPERIENCE OF THE ROOT CHAKRA

I never experienced the dramatic eruption of pranic energy (*udghata*) that occurred in Swami Kripalu's late thirties, which quickly activated his chakra system and relentlessly drove his spiritual evolution forward for the remainder of his life. Instead of a lightning bolt hurtling up the chakras, I'd liken the development of my subtle body to the growth of a flower rooted in the earth. As different facets of my being get freed up, it feels energetically that my yoga practice is readying me to bloom. That said, one experience of the chakras stands out in my memory.

In December 2001, I was given a month off from my normal duties to finish a first draft of the Kripalu Yoga book. Danna and I holed up in Woodstock, Vermont, where my sister had a second home, and settled into a retreat-like schedule. We greeted the day with postures, pranayama, and meditation. Then I'd write while Danna did her Kripalu Center marketing department work until lunch, after which we would take a long walk. Then came a second writing period for me, during which Danna edited my morning output and prepared our evening meal. We closed the work day with a few postures and time for *yoga nidra* (deep relaxation in corpse pose). At the end of relaxation, Danna needed a half-hour to finish dinner prep, so I started doing thirty minutes of *anuloma viloma* (alternate nostril breathing) to fill the void.

Two weeks passed uneventfully before an evening came when Danna predictably headed off to the kitchen. Starting pranayama, I quickly fell into a soothing rhythm and was startled when my peace was disturbed by an irritating noise. I thought it was a neighbor using a power tool in their adjoining backyard. But as I turned my attention to the sound, I was astonished to discover it coming from inside my body in the area of my sacrum. Without thinking, I focused my awareness there and immediately found myself internalized and gazing at a wedge-shaped structure, which was clearly where the vibration was coming from. It was a non-descript grey color that occurred to me as bone. And suddenly I was inside the structure and amazed to find it cavernous and covered with a velvety red material that looked and felt like the folds of a luxurious fabric.

The space was humming with a melodious, droning music that sounded part instrumental and part vocal. I was told intuitively that this was the Queen's chamber and the chant was being played and sung by her many attendants. There was a strong perfume-like fragrance, and the whole environment felt feminine and spilling over with female energy. I wondered who or what the Queen was, and what it would be like to meet her. In response, the attendants twittered with laughter, as if this was a preposterous thought, but I could not see them anywhere. Right then, even though my mind had not gone there, I felt a twinge of sexual arousal. As soon as it registered, I was ejected from the chamber and found myself back on my cushion, wondering what the heck had just happened. There was nothing to do but resume my pranayama until Danna came to get me for dinner.

The unusual nature of this experience stayed with me and led me to wonder if I had somehow entered the first or muladhara chakra. I had high hopes this might be the starting point for an energy awakening process in which I would experience each of the chakras in turn, but the remainder of our time in Woodstock passed uneventfully. Afterward, I went back to my desk job. I've long used the adhara points on a daily basis to move into meditation and have had other experiences of the chakras, a few of which proved inflexion points in my life, but nothing quite like this one.

I have described the energy centers as circular areas but that may cause a question to arise: Why do some yogic texts call them padmas or lotuses? Like a flower, an energy center can be closed or open. An inactive center is closed. An active center is open. A fully activated center blossoms into an energetic vortex and swirls like a whirlpool. It is logical that each energy center has a specific location in the subtle body and is reflexively linked to a physical nerve plexus and set of organs. But the texts describe each center as having a ruling god and goddess, a propitiating mantra, an element such as fire or water, a color, and a sacred geometric symbol. All of this is truly beyond comprehension. Many branches of ancient knowledge were compiled to produce these descriptions of the energy centers for use in various yogic rites. It is very difficult to understand them without personal experience. Even so, it is beneficial for a modern student to make a general acquaintance with these teachings.

BE A DISCERNING STUDENT

Swami Kripalu drew upon a multitude of yogic models, two of which are especially noteworthy. The chakra system as discussed here, and the five *koshas* (sheaths) presented in Chapter 11 of my prior book. While visually different, each maps the same territory by diagramming the gross and subtle levels of the human person. Where the koshas chart the journey to Self that is made by introverting awareness, the chakras are a template to arrive at the same destination through energy raising. Taken together, these two models have the potential to complement one another, with each being helpful in different types and stages of practice.

In the treatises of ancient yoga, descriptions of the various vital airs or pranic-flows are found. Hatha Yoga is only the most recent expression of these teachings. All forms of yoga seek to purify the channels of the subtle body then draw this prana back into its source. Prana that reaches that source can be called "atman." These two names for prana are very significant. In the beginning stages of yoga, prana is the aliveness of the outer sheaths of the body. In the middle stages, prana is the awake intelligence of the mind's inner sheaths. After achieving the beyond-mind state, prana is not other than the soul.

The yogis of old did not see the chakras as existing in the body of everyday people. They believed these spiritualizing centers were ritually-installed in the body of an aspirant through yogic initiation. Swami Kripalu was exerting a modernizing influence in teaching that the chakras lie dormant in everyone and physically correspond to the adrenals, testes or ovaries, pancreas, thymus, thyroid, pituitary, and pineal glands.

Contemporary spiritual teachers often attribute psychological qualities to each chakra. In this way of thinking, all of us start our life focused on survival with our energy coalesced in the lowest center. As we mature, especially if we are actively practicing yoga and meditation, the critical mass of our energy has the potential to move up the chakra system. This movement is credited for driving self-development, as it's thought the chakra we identify with and operate from determines our values and perspective on life. Many students find this view helpful, but resist any tendency to reduce the complex process of human development to a simple set of energy shifts. As SK said, lots of intentional actions are required *to make our dreams of growth a reality.*

The traditional texts include verses praising yoga as a panacea whose unwavering practice is powerful enough to remedy any problem. SK made similar statements, usually in a setting where his intention to inspire students was obvious. Teachings such as these taken out of context can lead a student to view spiritual practice as a cure-all. In today's world, it may be unwise or insufficient to rely solely upon the healing power of yoga. Your evolutionary journey may be better served by seeking out the help of medical experts to address health needs, and psychotherapists trained in modalities proven to resolve mental and emotional issues, especially in the early and middle stages of your practice.

APPLYING THIS CHAPTER IN PRACTICE

Individuals vary widely in their ability to sense the pulse of subtle energy that Swami Kripalu said *drives the spontaneous play of children.* By the time we're socialized and arrive at adulthood, most of us have grown unmindful of its movements. Some folks are born with an ability to feel its flow inside their bodies that never leaves them. It appears that a rare few possess a talent enabling them to see its working in others with a type of second sight.

While yoga can re-sensitize you to the inner dance of breath and energy, it is not necessary to see or feel this inner flow to deepen your practice. Simply stay attuned to the felt sense of the body and the gentle nudges, subtle shifts of feeling, and intuitive knowings that make you more responsive on and off the mat. Many yogis start out as skeptics and over time become energy believers, not through gaining any extraordinary faculties, but through the results they see manifest in their lives.

The six bodily chakras are the rungs on the ladder of yoga. Asana, pranayama, pratyahara, dharana, dhyana, and samadhi: these are the practices that activate them. "Activation" means the revitalization of the nerve plexus and bodily region associated with that chakra. It can be said that the practice of yoga proceeds as each chakra is activated by the primal energy with the highest states of meditation not occurring until the ajna chakra and its commanding nerve center situated midway between the two eye brows are fully developed. Above that is the thousand petalled chakra, wherein dwells the untainted Spirit, beyond all duality.

CHAPTER 4

THE KUNDALINI POWER

As the earth is the basis of all mountains, the kundalini power is the basis of all forms of yoga. The Hatha Yoga Pradipika declares: Only one who knows kundalini knows yoga. The Goraksha Paddhati situates kundalini in the lower regions of the body. Other texts assert that kundalini is the foundation of the three worlds. Some commentators say it has two coils, others three coils, and still others eight coils. Although there is a big difference in the words used, none of these scriptural verses are wrong. A yogic aspirant should allow them to be thought-provoking.

Without a doubt, the most intriguing component of the yogic body is the *kundalini shakti* or "coiled power," a reservoir of biological and psychospiritual energy symbolized as a sleeping serpent circled around the base of the spine. In many tantric yoga schools, kundalini is extolled as the secret power that underlies yoga's efficacy with every element of practice playing some role in bringing this dormant force to an optimal level of activity. When speaking to Westerners, Swami Kripalu referred to kundalini shakti as the *great primal power*. In his Sanskrit-to-English book glossaries, he defined it as the *supreme spiritual energy*. In the follow teaching, he uses an unusual term that I have found especially helpful, describing kundalini as the *evolutionary force*.[1]

Above the anus, below the navel, at the root of the male and female sexual organs, here lies the kundalini. The yogic texts

[1] Kundalini is a Sanskrit adjective meaning "coiled." Shakti means "feminine power," which in Tantric philosophy is the dynamic outpouring of Spirit that gives birth to material creation. All of yoga is energy-based, but its various schools can be roughly categorized as being either energy-raising or awareness-focusing. Both approaches are capable of activating kundalini and encouraging it to ascend the chakra system.

depict kundalini symbolically as a coiled snake, but we can think of it as the evolutionary force. The ancient rishis, the yogis of the Middle Ages, and adept yogis from the present age all experienced this great primal power. Yogis of the future will also experience it, because yoga is a science that works on the basis of the evolutionary force. What the ancients called ascension or transmutation should be taken to mean "the conscious evolution of the individual." In the body of most individuals, the evolutionary force is sleeping and its existence remains unsuspected, but it can be awakened through the systematic practice of yogic disciplines. It is through activating the evolutionary force, directly or indirectly, that the profound benefits of yoga are attained.

One thing is clear on the face of his teachings: kundalini and prana are not synonymous terms. Prana is the life energy linked to the breath that flows through the secondary and peripheral channels of the yogic body. It is the subtle fuel upon which the body-mind runs. Kundalini is a force of a greater magnitude that operates exclusively in the central channel, which explains why it is referred to by an altogether different name. If prana is likened to the stepped-down current running through a home's electrical circuitry to safely operate its lights and appliances, kundalini is the full-on voltage connecting its electrical panel to the power grid. That's why yoga practices are meant to be done within the supportive context of a healthy and holistic lifestyle, which helps safeguard practitioners from exceeding the capacity of their individual wiring.

Yoga books and teachers of our modern age equate the life energy of the body (prana) with the kundalini power. From the viewpoint of ancient yoga, this is incorrect. The life energy and kundalini power are different. Similarly, yoga practitioners—both male and female—assert that they experience the kundalini power when having sex. This gross observation is miles away from the truth. Yet from another viewpoint, there is some degree of validity in these remarks. The quickening of the life energy is a praiseworthy first step in yoga. Until it is taken, there is no way to arouse the sleeping kundalini power and make it upfacing (flow upward). For every adult human, the door of descent (downward flow) is always open.[2] *People do experience a reflection of kundalini in the sexual act, but only after it has been converted into enjoyment. This does not mean that their kundalini has been awakened or made upfacing, both of which only occur after the door of descent has been closed through ardent devotion and the door of ascent opened via yogic techniques.*

Quotes like these piqued my curiosity about this mysterious force that is meant to play a central role in yoga. In response, I set out to answer a simple three-word question: What is kundalini?

SURVEYING THE CONTEMPORARY LITERATURE

It was the early 1980s when I embarked on this inquiry. That was long before online searches and Amazon.com. But alternative bookstores carried a small selection of on-point paperbacks. Most were organized in a similar fashion. They opened with an emotionally gripping account of the author's awakening experience. Next came a middle section more-or-less parroting the models set out in the traditional yogic texts. They closed with speculations about the potential and perils of these teachings in the postmodern West, where it seemed the phenomenon of kundalini awakening was occurring with increased frequency.

While interesting reads, these books offered little practical guidance. Taken together, they left me feeling bewildered by this life-transforming energy that activates in a small subset of yoga and meditation practitioners, and sometimes in otherwise ordinary individuals without any apparent cause, to "rise up the spine and find expression in spiritual knowledge, mystical vision, psychic powers, and ultimately, enlightenment."[3] If kundalini really existed, I wanted to do everything possible to become one of those fortunate few.

[2] This sentence contrast humans with animals, who are only sexually active in seasonal periods of heat or rut.

[3] This statement is from Gopi Krishna (1903-83), an Indian householder who experienced a sudden energy awakening after years of early morning meditation. In 1971, he wrote *Kundalini: The Evolutionary Energy in Man*, a first-person account considered a spiritual classic, followed by sixteen other titles. For more on Gopi Krishna, see the footnote on page 49. Another representative book from that era is *The Kundalini Experience*, published in 1976 by Dr. Lee Sannella, a psychiatrist who studied and wrote about the kundalini phenomenon until his death in 2010.

I returned to the yogic texts hoping to find myself better positioned to apply their teachings in my practice. Yet even with this broader background their meaning remained shrouded in symbolism. It seemed my only recourse was to just keep doing the yoga I knew. At least Swami Kripalu was sensitive to my predicament:

> *Yogis become famous today by proclaiming that their kundalini has awakened. While they have genuinely experienced something they call awakening, that does not mean they have gained a real understanding of the kundalini power. Absent this understanding, their remarks will not have much value and run the risk of generating even greater confusion. The topic of kundalini is addressed in the Siva Samhita, Goraksha Paddhati, Gheranda Samhita, and Hatha Yoga Pradipika. These texts are valuable not because they are ancient but because they contain trustworthy guidance. Yet they are written in a way that requires a reader to have progressed through many preliminary stages of yoga practice to decode and properly interpret them. The traditional way for a student to remedy this problem is to run to their gurudev for answers, which enables the teacher to unlock the secrets of the texts by providing the keys at the opportune moment when the student is ready to put their teachings into practice. Using this correct approach, I have been able to resolve the mystery of kundalini for a few close disciples. Absent a competent teacher, a student needing answers to these questions is on the horns of a dilemma. Current writings are insufficient, but the ancient teachings cannot be understood.*

BREATHWORK

Right around that time, Danna and I signed up for a program at the original Kripalu Yoga Ashram in Sumneytown, Pennsylvania, called the Inner Quest Intensive. Three days of group yoga practice, structured personal growth work, social silence, and portion-controlled eating led into a culminating session called "breathwork." Entering the program room, blankets had been neatly laid out for all thirty participants. A contingent of extra staff appeared to serve as "breath coaches," each of whom would be responsible for a small group of "breathers." Sitting on our blankets, we were instructed in a technique called circular breathing. An energetic and full inhalation taken through the open mouth was immediately followed by a relaxing out-breath. Just before the exhalation completed, the next inbreath would be initiated, enabling the breath to flow in a dynamic fashion.

Placing our hands on our upper chest, we gave the technique a test drive to feel the powerful breathing pattern it produced. Then the session was explained by the leader in the simplest of terms. All the intensive participants were to lie on their blankets and get comfortable. Starting together, we would breathe in this active fashion for one hour, after which we would have time for relaxation. As I was getting situated, my breath coach introduced himself as an ashram resident named Ashok. He told our little group that he had done this form of breathwork many times and it was safe to give ourselves fully to the process. All we had to do was raise a hand and he would be there to respond to our needs.

Spirits were high as the breathing began, but after only a few minutes the group hit a collective wall. It felt impossible to continue breathing at this depth and pace. Wails and sobs could be heard throughout the room, but the microphoned leader urged us to stay focused and persevere with the breath. Soon something akin to a runner's second wind kicked in and things quieted down. Once that occurred, my awareness of everything happening around me was eclipsed by all sorts of inner sensations. A while later, a powerful energy began to stir in the core of my body that wanted to move and spread out but was blocked at various points that became painfully evident. My awareness was drawn into these dark places, triggering an array of poignant and forgotten memories, and compelling me to feel an almost unbearable degree of physical and emotional distress. Tears poured out of my eyes as I engaged in what felt like a life and death struggle.

Ashok came to my side and spoke directly into one ear, telling me to stay with the breath but make sure I was relaxing as much as possible on the exhale. I did my best to follow his instruction, but my breathing remained halting and labored. This heaving, while nothing close to the technique we'd been taught, was the best I could do. Right at the crisis point, when everything in me was instinctively fighting the process, the energy pushed through whatever had been obstructing it, and my body was permeated by an orgasmic bliss. Breathing became effortless, and alongside the euphoria I was overtaken by a mixture of relief and gratitude to have made it through the ordeal. When I returned my attention to the technique, I was able to ride the wave of the breath in a way heretofore unknown to me, and cycle through several build-ups and breakthroughs.

When the group was told to let the circular breath go, my time sense had entirely stopped working. It felt that we had been breathing forever, yet it also seemed the hour had passed in just a few minutes. I was cognizant enough of the outside world to hear the leader's instruction. But ceasing the circular breath was like stepping off some kind of internal cliff, and I free-fell into an alternate reality. In dreams and visions, I journeyed into a light-filled realm. Whether my trip ended in mystical union or deep sleep is hard to tell, but for a while all normal mentation ceased. Eventually my bodily awareness returned. Opening my eyes, I saw that almost everyone had left the room. Only Ashok and a few other stragglers remained, the rest of the group having gone to lunch. Assuring Ashok that I was okay alone, I stayed put for the better part of an hour, needing time to re-occupy my body and integrate everything that had just happened.

In the weeks that followed, I found myself asking whether the energy that had briefly become active in me was prana or kundalini. The early stages of the breathing process were marked by all sorts of tingling, inner currents, and unusual sensations. It made sense that these were the results of amplified prana. But the potent force stirred up in the end stages felt altogether different, and the amount of impactful psycho-emotional experience condensed into the time when it was active was hard to fathom. Only one thing was certain. Whatever propelled me forward on that journey from blockage to breakthrough was far more intelligent than my thinking mind.

Practicing yoga and meditation felt different after that breathwork session. I knew viscerally that hidden beneath the conscious surface of my body and mind was a primal energy that was both healing and evolutionary. It seemed self-evident that a regular posture and pranayama practice was meant to keep it freed up. Yet what this energy was, and how best to think about it, and continue to work with it, remained a mystery. In search of understanding, I returned to my yogic studies.[4]

KUNDALINI VIDYA

Eventually I found several contemporary yoga schools espousing slightly different takes on the traditional kundalini teachings. Each saw their lineage as carrying on the ancient *kundalini vidya* or "science of kundalini."[5] Philosophical systems often begin with a big picture view that links our human lives with the natural world in which we live. These lineages propound a cosmology—a theory explaining the origin of the universe and the role of human beings in it—grounded in the yogic conception of Brahman. Brahman is the unchanging Absolute, the supreme reality and ground of being that undergirds the material universe. While itself remaining unmanifest, Brahman is said to emanate an intelligent power (shakti) that creates, sustains, and continually evolves the constantly changing world we perceive with our mind and senses. On the level of the macrocosm, kundalini is described as *adi shakti* which means *the first force in creation* from which all the secondary forces of nature are derived. In this big picture perspective, kundalini is the primordial power and ordering intelligence that issues forth from the formless Brahman to give rise to the natural world.

These systems go on to explain how the same creative power that

[4] In the ashram, this form of breathwork was taught as a yogic kriya, which means "a practice that stimulates spontaneous healing actions," but it is not one of the traditional yogic pranayamas. It is a modern method of breathing that appears to have originated in the 1960s with an American teacher named Leonard Orr (1937-2019). Orr had studied yoga in India and called his innovative approach *Rebirthing*. Since then, many teachers have developed variants taught under different names. Readers wanting to learn more may benefit from the cogent intellectual view put forth by psychiatrist Stanislav Grof in *Holotropic Breathing*, and the artful guidance in doing the technique provided by Jim Leonard in *Vivation*.

[5] All these schools are organized around the traditional energy-based teachings and practices of yoga, Vedanta, and Tantra. I am presenting a synthesis here supported by SK quotes and excerpts. There are significant doctrinal differences among these schools. For example, one says the true seat of kundalini is in the brain with its activating trigger lying at the base of the spine. For more depth, see *A Systematic Course in the Ancient Tantric Techniques of Yoga and Kriya* by Swami Satyananda Saraswati published by the Bihar School of Yoga; *Kundalini Yoga* by Sri Swami Sivananda published by the Divine Life Society; and *Kundalini Vidya, The Science of Spiritual Transformation* by Joan Shivarpita Harrigan.

births the macrocosm (*samashti pind*) is at work within the microcosm of the human body (*vyashti pind*). In this view, kundalini activates at conception to initiate the organic process in the womb that establishes a template for the nervous system and accomplishes the myriad tasks associated with germinal, embryonic, and fetal development. When the fetus has grown to viability, a significant residue of kundalini energy remains, which coalesces at the base of its spine. After birth, the flowing currents of vital energy initiated in utero by kundalini are sustained by the breath and known as prana. It is this milder form of life energy that animates the body-mind when the kundalini power is said to be asleep.

Even in dormancy, kundalini continues to play a vital role in a person's well-being by providing a weighty energetic core that anchors their body-mind system in a healthy homeostasis. There are a few times when kundalini is known to interrupt its slumber, which are helpful pointers for yoga practitioners. During the rapid growth spurt that follows puberty, kundalini reactivates to bring adolescents to the peak of their vitality around the age of sixteen. It can also awaken when our survival is seriously threatened. In those moments, it is experienced as the high amplitude energy coursing through our system when the fight-or-flight response is powerfully triggered. Kundalini also stirs in times of sexual activity as the energy of procreation capable of sparking new life. In all these cases, it quickly goes back to sleep. It is said that kundalini awakens a final time in the dying process, when it uncoils to travel back up the spine and leave the body at the moment of death.[6]

[6] These ideas could help explain why surviving a serious trauma, or experiencing a Near Death Experience (NDE), can in some cases lead to a bioenergetic or spiritual awakening. The yoga tradition recognizes ten ways an adult's evolutionary energy can be active. 1. A fortuitous birth in which the kundalini energy remains active from childhood onward, or reactivates during adolescence as part of the maturation process and remains awake thereafter. 2. Aushadhi, activation through the ingestion of carefully-prepared herbs, which may have a rough parallel in our times with the use of traditional plant medicines and psychedelics. 3. Tapas, the ardent performance of purifying austerities. 4. Through japa, mantra meditation, and devotional chanting, which use the "sound current" or nada as the means of activation. 5. By the practice of pranayama alone. 6. Through the disciplined practice of Karma Yoga as taught in the Bhagavad Gita, or awareness-focusing Kriya Yoga as taught in the Yoga Sutra, or Raja Yoga as taught in various texts. 7. Through Hatha Yoga as taught in the Hatha Yoga Pradipika and similar energy-raising texts. 8. Through Tantric rituals, some of which generate overwhelming fear, invoke specific deities, or involve sexuality and other conduct that transgresses taboos and violates social norms. 9. By close or intimate contact with a person whose energy is awake, which traditionally means a

Often, I've been asked what happens when the kundalini strongly awakens. Some feel excited, some start shivering, some faint. Some begin to rock, others swing round and round using the buttocks as a pivot, some leap like a frog, some dance with abandon. Some chant mantras or sing loudly with great feeling, while others murmur, or cry, or laugh, or roar and scream. Some sit very still, or lie in trance, or fall into yogic sleep, or are transported into higher states of consciousness. Some bend forward, or bend backward, or twist the spine, or do other asanas and mudras known to yoga and remain in them for a long time. Some breathe fast, or deeply, hold the breath, or find their breath stopping of its own accord, or have other pranayamas occur spontaneously. Some have celestial visions, some have frightening visions, some see floods of light or vivid colors. Some lose control of urination; others witness the discharge of their semen. While these yogic experiences defy categorization, all of them can lead an aspirant into the mysterious realm of dhyana (depth meditation).

From the perspective of kundalini vidya, one purpose integrates all the disciplines of yoga, each of which in some way readies a practitioner to draw upon this reservoir of untapped energy to spark and spur on their growth and development. A healthy lifestyle builds the strong bodily container required to properly host the dormant kundalini. Right living (dharma) and the yogic practice of character building aligns the mind with the ethical principles (yama and niyama) innate to human nature, preparing the mind-based personality for a positive awakening. Asana coupled with the basic pranayamas begin the overt activation process. Together they open the gross body to greater aliveness, increasing the flow of prana through the subtle body to uplift physical health. A second set of cleansing pranayamas clears the inner channels of obstructions. These may be followed by vigorous pranayamas in which the breath is pumped then held long enough to trigger the fight or flight response and arouse the sleeping force. These energy-activating breathing practices often include mantras, mudras, and visualizations that focus attention

transmission from guru to disciple through physical touch, speech, glance, or directed thought called *shaktipat diksha.* 10. Through Ishvara Pranidhana, the profound surrender of the individual will to God or one's higher self.

on the body's core, where kundalini is said to be sleeping, and direct it to enter the central channel. Paradoxically, other yoga schools couple an attitude of surrender and non-effort with the practice of pacifying pranayamas done in concert with mantras and other meditative techniques that slow the respiration rate until the faint flow of breath seems to stop entirely, a non-volitional experience called "breath suspension" that can also activate the kundalini.[7]

The coil-shaped kundalini lies with its head lowered in slumber, obstructing the doorway to the Absolute (Brahmadvara.) It is only when kundalini awakens and lifts its head that the entryway into mystical yoga is revealed. Most seekers must religiously practice asana, pranayama, and pratyahara (methodically drawing the attention inward) to purify the body and mind sufficiently for kundalini to awaken. My guru lovingly placed his hand upon my head, gracing me with shaktipat diksha (the yogic initiation that quickly activates kundalini). The first task of the awakened kundalini is to enter this doorway to unclog the lower portion of the central channel, and then proceed upward to pierce the granthis. It is only after this is done that the life energies (prana together with its counterpart apana) can flow freely in the central channel. It is these ascending energies that enliven the chakras and enable the mind (citta) to become absorbed in meditation.

Yoga's model of the subtle body allows the advent of a strong kundalini awakening to be visually depicted. Stirring from its slumber, the coiled serpent raises its head, exposing the lower opening of the central channel. Entering into what the yogis imagined was a thin hollow core of the spinal column, the lightning-like kundalini uncoils to clear its major blocks. Prana is now able to enter on the heels of kundalini and begin its ascent, which activates the chakra system and generates a wide-range

[7] The descriptions in this paragraph are oriented to the body-based approach of hatha yoga and other energy-raising yoga systems. It is also known that intensive mental concentration as practiced in the awareness-focusing systems, or heartfelt devotion and surrender to a higher power as practiced in bhakti yoga, are equally capable of rousing the sleeping kundalini. SK attributed his awakening to his guru's touch (shaktipat diskha) and not any of these willful practices – see Chapter 4 of *Dharma Then Moksha*.

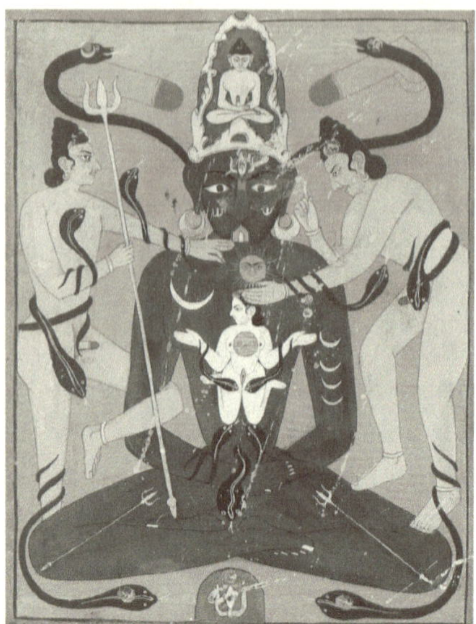

An eighteenth-century painting by an unknown Tantric artist depicting the traditional symbolism associated with a yogi's Kundalini awakening.
Source: Wiki Commons.

of spontaneous actions (kriyas and mudras) that untie the three knots (granthis) and clear the system of localized blocks (marmans).[8] These actions and the internal urges prompting them produce sensations that draw the attention inward and upward, quieting the outer-directed senses, and absorbing the yogi in a dynamic form of introspective meditation. This coming together of the evolutionary force, the life energy of the body, and focused mental awareness reflects an all-out attempt of an individuated soul to regain consciousness of its spiritual source in the Absolute. Many contemporary writers describe the process of kundalini awakening as an event that happens quickly or even effortlessly. SK was of a decidedly different opinion.

After kundalini activates, a seeker must meditate regularly for years to complete the awakening process. At first, they are likely to face strong sensual desires, both physically and mentally, as their whole body is set alight with passion. Practicing yoga in the midst of these desires is a formidable task, but one who ceases to practice will find their energy descending into unconsciousness. Those able to persevere will become aware of the granthis (knots or nerve tangles) that exist in the subtle body and then experience the slow process of the chakras flowering. But this cannot happen if one is full of energy-blocking impurities. Most seekers find that asana and pranayama practice must continue to sufficiently purify the body and

[8] This aggressive opening and unclogging of the lower channel is exclusive to the renunciate model of kundalini awakening. Individuals who have undergone it report a rapid purging of the physical body and parallel disgorging of unconscious material from the mind. In the householder model, purification happens gradually.

mind. Without this hatha (bodily) yoga, one does not find the motivation to practice raja yoga (meditation) intensively. While each person's path will be different, a seeker should not expect to quickly or easily reach yoga's higher stages.

Reading his books and transcripts closely, I could see that his teachings were not entirely at loggerheads with the contemporary accounts I had read. SK agreed that the *first stirrings* of kundalini could be sudden and spontaneous. But experience had taught him that these initial awakenings must be followed by a mix of body-based practices to keep the energy flowing, together with introspective and devotional techniques that heal emotional blocks and resolve psychological issues, either of which can prevent kundalini from rising into the upper chakras. This made me wonder if many of these contemporary reports reflected an initial awakening where an opportunity to cultivate a more far-reaching developmental process might have been missed.

He also seemed to be saying that a kundalini awakening could not only stall, but stagnate, and even bring harmful consequences, something I was unable to understand at the time but would come to appreciate later:

A sadhak must remain aware that awakening the primal power is one thing and making it move upward is something else entirely. Kundalini's rightful purpose is to help a yogi advance toward samadhi. Other uses will result in regression or downfall. Anyone ceasing to practice is likely to find their inspiration coming to an end. While continued efforts may keep the kundalini active, those departing from dharma (healthy lifestyle, morality, and ethical restraints) will eventually fall prey to adharma and its many vices. Most simply abandon the path, but some become diseased or mad. It is delusion to assume the role of a teacher at this stage, and those who do are likely to proceed down a wrong path. A sincere practitioner swiftly progresses to a point where the line between pleasure-seeking and spirituality becomes thin. Indulging the senses to the point of excess stifles the process, which challenges them to practice moderation. Overly identifying with one's talents, charisma, and acclaim is the next threshold that must be crossed. Those progressing further may fall prey to the allure of extraordinary abilities, as it is easy to become a slave of these siddhis (psychic powers). A full kundalini awakening presents these well-known pitfalls. Only a pure-minded yogi displaying great courage can navigate them.

A yogi walking this path of post-awakening practice discovers that their experience of kundalini does not remain static. They learn the important lesson that kundalini is a primordial force and should not be mistaken for any of its levels or expressions. In the root chakra, it is the fierceness of the survival instinct. In the second chakra, it is compulsive sexuality and lust. In the third chakra, it is blind self-interest and the drive for security and power. Together these unconscious drives reflect what Swami Kripalu called the *gross kundalini.* No matter how seemingly problematic, all of these drives are essential for life. None of their energies can be denied or suppressed for long. Instead, they must be sublimated into their healthy and higher expressions.

In the fourth chakra, kundalini expresses as empathy and love. In the fifth, it takes the form of creative and often artistic expression. In the sixth chakra, it's the intuitive capacity and intellectual brilliance underlying genius and visionary leadership. In the seventh chakra, it is a continually self-surpassing consciousness that has the potential to culminate in a state some researchers have labelled "absolute unitary being."[9] These sublime expressions are what he called the *subtle kundalini.* Aware of this spectrum, the yogis of old taught that a well-orchestrated kundalini awakening can be trusted to catalyze an organic growth process that reliably leads a practitioner to self-discovery and beyond.

[9] Absolute Unitary Being is a term coined by the medical doctors and pioneering contemplative researchers Andrew B. Newberg and Eugene G. d'Aquili to describe the highest mystical state that tracks closely with the teachings of yoga. See *Why God Won't Go Away, The Biology of Belief.* While absorbed in my study of kundalini vidya, I was taken by the apparent newness of its ideas. But eventually I concluded that it was not that different from the theology of my Catholic upbringing. God the Father is transcendent of creation, which is permeated by the Holy Spirit, the power through which the will of God acts. This divine power is fully expressed in the incarnate son, who represents our highest potential. Some progressive religious commentators have pointed out the similarities between the energetic benediction received by the twelve disciples on the day of Pentecost with the yogic teachings on kundalini awakening. At first the disciples saw visions and spoke in tongues, but eventually their awakening matured into the higher capacities that these once-ordinary individual displayed as the first ministers of the Christian gospel.

At this point, I finally felt able to formulate an intellectually sound answer to my question: What is kundalini? In yoga philosophy, kundalini is the cosmic force that brings each of us and everything in the natural world into being. It is the pure creative potential from which existence takes shape. In yoga practice, kundalini is a drop of that potential expressing as the primal energy underlying your being, which is both the taproot of your life force as an individual, and the essence of ultimate reality that you aspire to know through meditation.

Suddenly, I understood a cryptic statement made by Swami Kripalu that heretofore was undecipherable: *Divine contact can only be had through kundalini.* The logic of this was now apparent. Kundalini shakti is what links the transcendent Absolute to all the relative dimensions and individual expressions of reality. Whether you seek to know it through bodily yoga and energy-raising breathwork, awareness-focusing meditation, devotional rituals, self-inquiry, or other practices is a secondary consideration. If like SK, you accept yogic philosophy and its model of the subtle body, kundalini flowing upward through the conduit of the central channel is the only route back to your spiritual source.

It is a rare yogi who knows what kundalini is. Acquainting a yogic aspirant with kundalini is more difficult than helping a person blind from birth understand the color spectrum, or a deaf person the range of musical notes. As in these examples, kundalini has many forms. But its two basic forms of subtle and gross are inclusive of all. The gross kundalini operates as the animal energies of the lower chakras, which must be respected. The subtle kundalini operates as the higher energies of the upper chakras through which superior states of heart and mind are realized. Those who know yoga propitiate kundalini in both of its conjoined forms, transmuting its gross power into increasingly subtle energies through dhyana (meditation), then sublimating both into samadhi (unity consciousness).

BE A DISCERNING STUDENT

There is no easy way to explain yoga's millennial-old model of kundalini awakening in the terminology of contemporary science. The two arise from entirely different worldviews. Yet it is well-known that mental health professionals regularly encounter clients troubled by kundalini-like symptoms. Leading members of the American Psychological Association (APA) are actively debating how clinicians should respond in terms of effective treatment. Progressive advocates, mostly from the field of Transpersonal Psychology, have lobbied to add a category of "kundalini syndrome" to *The Diagnostic and Statistical Manual of Mental Disorders* (DSM), the handbook used worldwide to diagnose patients presenting mental health issues. They proposed this new category to offset the tendency of uninformed physicians and psychologists to pathologize individuals who may be transitioning into healthy post-conventional states of human development, and who will stabilize if given supportive care.

The current fifth edition of the DSM does not include this category. Apparently, that's because clarity is lacking on the underlying causes of the kundalini process in medical terms. But as a result of the debate, there is growing consensus on a list of commonly-reported motor, somatosensory, audiovisual, and mental symptoms, which closely correspond to experiences well-known and documented in the yoga tradition.[10] Also noteworthy is the inclusion starting with the fourth DSM edition of the diagnostic category of "Qigong Psychotic Reaction" among its "glossary

[10] Here are some of the recognized symptoms of the proposed DSM category "kundalini syndrome." Motor: Spontaneous and involuntary movements including muscle twitches, jerks, or spasms. Body shakes, vibrates, trembles, or assumes yogic or other positions, and may freeze or lock into those positions for no apparent reason. Abnormally slow or rapid heart rate. Breathing may spontaneously stop, or its pace may become rapid, shallow, or deep. Somatosensory: Pains in specific parts of the body that start and stop abruptly. Headaches or feeling of cranial pressure. Extreme sensations of heat or cold moving through the body. Itching, prickling, tingling, stinging, or crawling sensations. Awareness of energy currents rushing, circulating, or discharging through the body. Physical sensations starting in the lower body and moving up to the head, often along the spine, and in some cases back down to the abdomen. Spontaneous ecstatic and orgasmic feelings. Audiovisual: Hearing inner sounds such as whistling, hissing, chirping, roaring, waterfalls, or musical instruments like bells, drums, or flutes. Seeing internal lights, colors, or geometric patterns. Synesthesia, especially experiencing energy as sound currents or flowing light. Mental: Sudden states of intense fear, anxiety, depression, hatred, or confusion. Sudden states of ecstasy, bliss, peace, love, devotion, joy, or cosmic unity. Thoughts speeding up, slowing down, or stopping altogether. Observing one's thoughts and feelings as if a bystander or falling into trance. Experiencing oneself as larger than the physical body. Expanded or otherwise non-ordinary states of consciousness that may be accompanied by revelatory or transformative insights.

of culture-bound syndromes." QPR is described as a time-limited condition appearing in individuals who become overly involved in practices such as Chinese Qigong, Indian yoga, or Buddhist meditation and are observed to lose touch with reality.

All of this activity on the part of the APA suggests there is something objectively real in the phenomenon of kundalini awakening. If that's correct, yoga's claim that the *great primal power* can be activated for the purposes of growth and evolution may have merit. How then is an aspiring yoga student to proceed? In Swami Kripalu's mind, that depends upon whether you are a renunciate or a householder.

Yoga is a science, but it is a mystical science. And at the center of all those mysteries is kundalini shakti. A spiritual aspirant practicing yoga will find that certain questions arise in the mind from their process of inner growth. At first these seem to be a long list of entirely different questions. Eventually it becomes clear that there are only a few fundamental questions with progressively deepening solutions. The answer to a first level question is useful for that level only. In the second level, the question takes a slightly different form. The first level solution becomes useless, and the second level answer must be found. Only after faithfully practicing for many years and reaching yoga's climax is the secret behind this mystery revealed. For all these years, it is kundalini that has been evolving both the question and the solution to bestow liberating knowledge upon the aspirant.

CHAPTER 5

THE TWO PATHS

Wrong notions about kundalini have become so firmly established in society that it may be impossible to remove them. Ignoring this confusion, kundalini comes unbidden onto the path of faithful yoga practitioners, and it is from that point they progress spiritually.

Swami Kripalu's perspective on how yoga practice is meant to activate the *great primal power* stands alone among all the teachers, texts, and teachings I've studied. One defining principle differentiates his view, the significance of which cannot be overstated. The kundalini power can be awakened in either one of two ways. The first is *quickly and completely*. The second is *gradually and partially*. It is these two types of kundalini awakening—complete and partial—along with the lifestyles and mindsets necessary to sustain them over time, that lie at the heart of SK's renunciate and householder paths.

In the ashram, it was generally thought the only genuine kundalini awakening was a strong one evidenced by a cluster of the symptoms referenced in Swami Kripalu's renunciate teachings, many of which are now mirrored in the DSM. On closer inspection, I don't believe this reflects the nuanced nature of his guidance to householders.

In both renunciate yoga and householder yoga, it is necessary to awaken the evolutionary force. Without this, it is not possible to develop spiritually. Renunciates are initiated into yoga and immerse themselves in its practice to swiftly and fully awaken the kundalini power. This method allows for rapid progress, but a renunciate yogi who fails to withdraw from the world encounters countless difficulties and soon discovers they cannot remain a traveler on this path. In householder yoga, the kundalini is awakened in its partial and tolerable form by doing practices that amplify the life force (prana). This protects the householder's physical health and mental stability, enabling them to practice yoga while living an active life in society. A dedicated householder welcoming the gradual purification and growth this approach brings will gain readiness and enter the stage of kundalini awakening without special initiation.

How can a householder realize the deeper potentials of yoga that Swami Kripalu says are only gained by activating the kundalini power without falling prey to its perils? Answering that question with the rigor required to actually practice it requires contrasting a householder kundalini awakening with the better-known version sought by renunciates.

COMPLETE AWAKENINGS

Each year some number of yoga practitioners, meditators, and otherwise ordinary people report symptoms consistent with the yogic definition of a strong kundalini awakening. Judging from their anecdotal reports, some suffer through a dreadful and disorienting time, while others derive great benefit. But few develop into anything akin to the yogic ideal of a saint or spiritual master. SK's teachings explain that a strong initial awakening is only the first of several factors that must come together to make for a *complete kundalini awakening.*

What makes renunciate yoga unique is that it quickly awakens the evolutionary force in its complete, uncontrollable, and furious form. Confronting its superior power, the mind becomes unstable, terrified, and prone to delusions. A strong awakening has the potential to transform a highly-fit aspirant into a great yogi, but on this path there is an indispensable need for a guru able to provide the initiations and ongoing guidance required to progress along it. Any such guru will only provide these initiations to a qualified disciple, meaning one who surrenders wholeheartedly to instruction; who agrees to live in seclusion; and who vows to practice yoga and only yoga for the rest of their life. It is foolhardy to strive to fully awaken the evolutionary force while continuing to live in society and harbor desires for wealth, pleasure, and notoriety. The texts warn us that one attempting this will fail on both accounts and gain neither human fulfillment nor spiritual liberation. I was the only disciple to whom my guru gave this initiation. At the time, I could not fathom why he was not initiating others. Now, through my own experience, I have come to understand.

In rare instances when all four of these conditions come together—a strong awakening, access to a genuine expert, the opportunity to live in a sheltered environment free from the need to earn a living or maintain a family, and an unwavering commitment to continual practice—the activated kundalini can drive a renunciate yogi forward in a rapid and relentless process of inner transformation. Swami Kripalu experienced this kind of awakening at age thirty-eight and afterward stayed true to his lifelong vows. An illustrated account of what that looks like appears in *Dharma Then Moksha*. In the above teaching, SK emphasizes the importance of *initiations*, which are instructions in esoteric or secret techniques that quickly arouse the kundalini power to full activity. These techniques are an essential element of renunciate kundalini yoga because they alone make its daily practice possible. Without them, a strong initial awakening will almost always fade out.[1]

Swami Kripalu's life story follows the arc of many Indian kundalini masters. He was sought out by an enigmatic guru at a young age and schooled in yoga's foundational teachings. After practicing those teachings for two decades and developing into an accomplished adult, his guru appeared in a vison and said *the time is right for you to commence your intensive practice.* Accepting this instruction, he ceased all his other activities, observing celibacy, eating a spartan diet, and practicing an

[1] These techniques are kept secret for two reasons. First, because they would be a distraction to the majority of yoga practitioners who are householders. Secondly, because they pose a risk of harm to unprepared practitioners and others lacking a qualified teacher. Verse 3.111 of the Hatha Yoga Pradipika is a text reference to one such technique written in a veiled way that cannot be interpreted by the uninitiated. A noteworthy difference between a complete renunciate and partial householder awakening is the way energy is described as rising. In response to the arousing renunciate techniques, the gross kundalini energy struggles to forcibly flow up the center of the spinal column, a process that may take years to culminate. In a partial awakening, the energy builds and gradually ascends the chakra system aided by regular meditation, but often without any overly strong sense of an upward flow.

energy-activating pranayama in four sittings totaling six hours a day for several months in succession. When his kundalini strongly awakened, his students and devotees were willing to support him in a lifestyle in which he ate one meal a day, spoke sparingly, studied scripture, and practiced yogic meditation ten hours every day for the next thirty years.[2]

If you as a reader find yourself blessed with all four of these factors—each of which is required to tolerate the long-term energetic and emotional volatility of renunciate-level practice without in some way acting out—my counsel mirrors the advice of Swami Kripalu: follow the guidance of your guru.

Lacking these factors, my way forward on his householder path felt anything but clear. I was certain he was pointing to some less-dramatic form of kundalini awakening that could be sustained by a householder yogi. Believing this issue stood between me and the higher stages of

[2] I've found it edifying to compare SK's experience with that of other modern yogis who had strong kundalini awakenings but lacked one or more of these four factors. Here are two examples. The previously mentioned author, Gopi Krishna, had a sudden kundalini awakening at age thirty-four after seventeen years of practicing a concentration-based form of meditation for three hours every morning outside of any religious tradition or teaching lineage. Lacking any post-awakening guidance, he spent a dozen years trying to stabilize his condition. At times he teetered on the edge of life and death, enduring unbearable heat in his body, and the mental extremes of ecstasy and depression. During these periods, he was unable to work and cared for by his wife. Eventually his condition did stabilize and the benefits of his kundalini awakening came to fruition. This allowed him to diagnose the cause of his awakening gone awry, which he attributed to the kundalini energy trying to ascend through the solar or heating nadi instead of the central channel. In the last three decades of his life, he became a respected writer, poet, social reformer, and advocate for women's rights, greatly admired for his unique blend of genuine humility and visionary genius. The American yogi, Franklin Albert Jones, studied with several kundalini adepts in the late 1960s including Swami Muktananda. After a strong awakening, his connection to any lineage or external guidance frayed, and he became a popular teacher living at the center of a large California ashram community and espousing his own highly non-traditional brand of kundalini yoga. While by all accounts a powerful individual who radiated tremendous energy, as well as a brilliant speaker and prolific author, his life was marked by a sense of grandiosity that led him to adopt a series of spiritual names including Bubba Free John, Da Free John, Da Love-Ananda, Da Avabhasa, and Adi Da Love-Ananda Samraj, each suggestive of a higher spiritual status. He also displayed a behavioral licentiousness that spawned moral controversy, much of which concerned his sexualizing of students. The life stories of both individuals synopsized above are rich with detail as reflected in their autobiographies: *Living with Kundalini* (Gopi Krishna) and *The Knee of Listening* (Adi Da). Extending this kind of analysis to other individuals, you are likely to find that kundalini is a strong energy that often brings out these kind of extremes in people.

yoga, I was determined to resolve it, but all I could do was follow his instruction to *just keep practicing.*

In the body of most human beings, the evolutionary force is entirely dormant and can rightly be described as "sleeping." When the evolutionary force awakens in its complete form, primal energy surges through the system leaving no doubt that the evolutionary force has ended its slumber. But when kundalini awakens in its partial form, there may be few if any indicators, and it can easily be thought to still be sleeping. A partial awakening gradually transforms an ordinary person into an unusually gifted and creative individual. The great yogis knew from experience that the fountainhead of all such talents is the evolutionary force. That is why they described the kundalini of these gifted individuals as "partially awake." While this form of awakening is best pursued through the systematic practice of yoga, it can also occur through the steadfast observance of good habits and the rules appropriate to a particular religious faith, artistic medium, branch of science, or other field of activity. Even if a brilliant scientist or passionate artist does not know yoga at all, their devotion to excellence makes them into a fit yogic aspirant, and partially awakens their kundalini.

AN OPPORTUNITY PRESENTS

Looking back, I held tight to the ashram's model of a complete kundalini awakening far too long. It was tantalizing to imagine that some other-worldly energy was slumbering inside me that yoga might wake up to a level of activity that would whisk away my problems. Convinced I was falling short on the self-discipline needed to forcibly arouse my snoring kundalini, my response to everything became a knee-jerk "just practice harder."

An opportunity to move beyond this limiting model presented itself when I was invited to deliver the closing keynote talk at the 2007 yoga teacher's conference hosted by Vandita Kate Marchiesello. Vandita was a resident during the four years SK lived in the Pennsylvania ashram. After becoming an administrative leader and top-notch yoga teacher, she went on to apply the values SK held dear while married and raising a family of three. Vandita asked me to offer a retrospective on the ashram experience. Wanting to do right by her, I spent two months researching American religious history to better understand the contemporary yoga movement. Everything I was learning led me to see the rise and fall of the Kripalu Center ashram as a continuation of the same societal forces that a century earlier had produced Emerson, Thoreau, and the American Transcendentalists. Journeying further back in time, I became fascinated by the Quakers and Shakers. Both of these early groups were known to tremble under the power of the holy spirit, a bodily experience they felt signaled a rebirth of the soul.

With the date of the keynote fast approaching, I engaged in a form of procrastination that drives Danna nuts. Instead of buckling down to finish the talk, I doggedly traced the legacy of the Quakers and Shakers forward in time. I found Pentecostal denominations attesting to the power of "spiritual quickenings" and affirming the place of ecstatic singing, vocal praising, joyous dancing, swaying, shouting, shaking, and even rolling on the floor in church services.[3] Alongside them were Charismatic Christians bearing witness to a similar experience of "being filled with the Holy Spirit," an emotionally-moving encounter with the divine said to result in miraculous healings and the gifts of prophecy and speaking in tongues. Even the progressive Unity School of Christianity acknowledged the role of these quickenings as "inflows of divine vitality that stir the soul to life and have the power to transform every level of a person's being." None of these groups saw spiritual quickening as the culmination of a person's faith journey. Much to the contrary, it was a "baptism of fire" that had to be kept burning bright through regular prayer, devotional worship, Bible study, and religious fellowship.

Mulling over this material brought to mind an encounter that happened in my college years. I was hitchhiking to see a girlfriend in Tuscaloosa, Alabama, and got dropped off in the middle of nowhere. First came a downpour, then a dramatic rise in temperature. Gradually it became obvious that no one was going to pick up this visibly steaming

[3] Holy roller is a term that arose in the 1800s to describe the most animated of these Protestant Christians. Initially, and often today when used by outsiders, the term is pejorative. When used by insiders to describe themselves, it is embraced as a badge of honor.

vagabond, and I passed the night under a bridge abutment. Early the next morning, an oversized Lincoln Continental pulled over. Climbing in the back, I was warmly greeted by the driver, a middle-aged lady whom I thanked profusely. A second woman sitting next to her turned to look at me but remained silent. The frowning man in the passenger seat was obviously not happy. Once on the road, he adjusted the sun visor and then its vanity mirror to keep an eye on me.

Settling into the big backseat, I noticed it was strewn with religious tracts that resembled comic books. They all orbited around a single theme, the importance of becoming spirit-filled. The best hitchhiking etiquette is to remain silent, which I did for a while, but eventually curiosity got the better of me. When I asked about these books and the experience of being spirit-filled, the driver was quick to respond and her words conveyed real conviction, "Don't think belief alone will save you. It's not enough to mouth the magic words, "I accept Jesus Christ into my heart as my Lord and Savior. That's a false teaching."

I'd encountered fundamentalists before, but something about this woman felt different. Along with her strident beliefs, she had an energy and brightness that commanded my attention. The woman continued, "Yes, you have to sincerely want the Lord, but you've got a brain. Think about it. No belief or act of your own can save yourself. You can only be saved by grace. When the Holy Spirit enters into you, that's the sign you've been saved. If that occurs, you will feel it for yourself, and won't need anyone else to tell you so. The Holy Spirit is God's active force. It alone gives you the power to live a Godly life. That's what it means to be spirit-filled."

There was a directness to this woman impossible not to respect. I didn't have an immediate reply, and for a time her bold proclamation hung in the air. The silence allowed a single line of thought to come clear in my mind, which I voiced, "I agree with you. Beliefs and words are not enough." Sensing something sincere in my response, she asked, "If that's true, what are you going to do about it?" Again, I didn't have an answer.

After a while, she instructed me, "When you get back home, find a spirit-filled church. Don't trust the label. You'll be able to feel it in the worship, in the music, in the congregation. If you are willing and open, the Spirit will seek you out, but you'll still need a good church to keep it alive in you." The conversation ended there, but I stepped out of that car feeling this woman had found a way to connect with some source of energy that was real for her. On top of this, it seemed the churches she frequented had found ways to not only spark this experience in new members but keep it active in their congregations. While I never felt called to act on her advice, it wasn't all that long before I found and joined the ashram.

Ordinary religion is outward-looking and aims to improve society. But there is also an inner-directed religion that seeks to rouse the spirit of individuals and spur on their growth. The speech, behavior, and positive mood displayed by someone animated by this moving spirit attracts the attention of other people. Often have I thanked All Merciful God for gracing me with many such high-spirited companions.

AN ALTERNATIVE MODEL COMES TO MIND

I couldn't point to anything definite I had gained by this line of extracurricular research, or the distant memory that had surfaced in its wake. None of it was salient enough to place front and center in my talk. With the conference only a week away, I acknowledged Danna's consternation and got busy. It took a day or two but I was able to trim my content to fit the time allotted and write an inspiring close to the talk.

The keynote was a joint effort, my talk spiced up by Danna's poetry. The Sunday morning we presented to an audience overspilling Kripalu Center's Main Chapel still shines in my mind as a cherished memory. Back home and relieved to have the pressure off, my mind returned to the topic of these quickenings and the things done by the denominations organized around them to keep the spirit active. That led me to think of our years as ashram residents and the high-energy chanting and dancing the community did daily. Connecting these dots, it became clear that my trip down that rabbit hole of research was no mistake. It was my interest in the Quakers and Shakers, and the seemingly senseless foray into charismatic Christianity that followed on its heels, that was now enabling me to see Swami Kripalu's teachings on partial kundalini awakenings in a whole new light.

It was a hoot to think of my ashram brothers and sisters as being spirit-filled. Yet I felt certain that Swami Kripalu was pointing to something very much along those lines in his householder teachings. Differing so markedly from the prevailing notion of a kundalini awakening, the similarities of these two known phenomena was easy to miss. But forging that link in my mind was tremendously important. If kept vital by ongoing practice and supportive lifestyle, the teachings of Swami Kripalu were clear. This more-manageable type of energy awakening could not only fuel a householder's personal growth but carry them up the ladder of yoga.

Anyone earnestly wanting to evolve to higher levels has to accept the help of kundalini. Complete awakenings are only for renunciate seekers of liberation. Does this mean men and women of the world have no possibility of evolving spiritually? No, that is an incorrect interpretation. Although kundalini usually lies dormant, it can become active in the human body in different forms. Instead of sleeping, it may become slightly active, or somewhat active, or obviously active. All of these I call partial activations.

CHAPTER 6

KUNDALINI AWAKENING FOR HOUSEHOLDERS

It is foolish to think the profound benefits of yoga can be gained without exercising the self-discipline required to partially awaken the evolutionary force and keep it continually active. This is how all energetic, brilliant, and talented men and women rise to worldly acclaim. Yoga emphasizes learning and exercising self-control because that's what keeps the evolutionary force active. A householder yogi understanding this secret can use it to advance toward Self-realization.

Looking back, I believe the ashram's greatest triumph was its ability to carry all sorts of ordinary people across the threshold of a partial kundalini awakening. Anyone dedicating a year or more to ashram residency went through a bootcamp-like training in which they did enough bodily yoga and pranayama to activate their primal energy. Eating a healthy diet and living the early-to-bed and early-to-rise ashram lifestyle, most new residents experienced a healing crisis of some kind and emerged out the other side decidedly more vibrant. This explains why so many young people coming for a relatively short volunteer stint opted to stay on and join the staff. It also suggests why so many older individuals and married couples with established family and professional lives became repeat guests. Something about the place was raising everyone's energy, and along with it their sense of aliveness and meaning.

In those early ashram years, Kripalu Center was a magnet and the energy I'm describing was palpable. It radiated from the staff. And the extended community, which included many former residents and regular guests, was full of bright, good humored, creative, and enterprising people. These are exactly the kind of yogis that Swami Kripalu's householder path was designed to produce.

This triumphant observation of mine is tinged with a bit of sadness as the community didn't have a model of yoga practice that recognized this great accomplishment. Measuring ourselves against the renunciate ideal of a complete kundalini awakening, ex-residents often felt like ashram dropouts. Even long-term residents playing leadership roles were at risk of seeing themselves as yogic failures. Instead of inspiring us to keep progressing along what for almost everyone was a householder path, this model hindered growth and often truncated our practices. That's why this chapter provides an alternative view.

My guidance to aspiring householders wanting to awaken kundalini in its partial form is to steadfastly practice the basic techniques of an established yoga system for a year-and-a-quarter.[1] *After this period of intensive practice, they should continue their yoga faithfully while pursuing their aims in life, but any activation that results must be kept in line with their duties and life circumstances through monitoring the duration and intensity of their practice. My experience is that a householder who perseveres like this in performing even the simplest techniques of yoga, if done properly and with full attention, can trust that they will appropriately awaken the evolutionary force.*

SAME GOAL, DIFFERENT PROCESSES

Right from the outset, it's important to know the guiding goal of renunciate and householder yoga practice with regards to kundalini awakening is one and the same. Both approaches seek to result in an enlivened chakra system functioning as an integrated whole. But the pathway taken to advance toward that common goal is markedly different.

Swami Kripalu described renunciate yoga as a *battle of prana and apana*. Prana is the ascending life force that yoga sees as wanting to

[1] Swami Kripalu was personally schooled by his guru over a 15-month period. As a teacher, he prescribed this same period of time for his students to practice any significant spiritual discipline. For more, see *Dharma Then Moksha*, pages 34-43.

elevate consciousness and surpass its current level of development. In Ayurvedic medicine, prana is the energy that brings new life into the system and carries nutrients into the cells. Apana is prana's counterbalance, the descending life force that wants to remain comfortable, pleasure itself when possible, and regress to the known and habitual. In Ayurveda, apana carries wastes out of the cells and body. A renunciate initiates this battle between prana and apana by engaging the kundalini power in its gross form as sexual energy. As the battle rages on, the chakra system is activated from bottom to top.

Whenever somebody starts the practice of renunciate yoga, they declare war on lust. They only fight this one battle, because they know that if they can win it, success on all other fronts will come. Prana is the hero, the life energy residing in the heart that wants to flow up to victory. Apana is the demon, the eliminative energy that resides in the sexual organs and wants to flow down and out to experience pleasure. The prana uses all its force to pull apana into the heart chakra. The apana uses all its force to resist and descend back into its resting place. In the beginning, the sleeping kundalini power is allied with apana and it remains victorious. If prana does not abandon its efforts, it grows strong enough to awaken kundalini. Eventually this enables prana to succeed in pulling apana up into the heart and higher centers, but time and time again this seeming victory does not prove steady, and apana soon descends. This is a very, very difficult path.

SK characterized householder yoga differently, as a *path of gradual purification and growth.* A householder walks this path by creating a lifestyle that supports good health and slowly but steadily raises prana to higher levels of activity. As energy builds, the ascending prana slowly ratchets up the chakra system, activating each center in turn. Much of this activity happens off the screen of conscious awareness, but sooner or later its long-term effects become discernible.

In India there are two religions. The religion of the recluse who wants immediate spiritual progress, and the religion of the householder living in society that is done alongside one's everyday duties.

A householder must first progress to physical health, mental tranquility, and a disposition of happiness. That much is needed for worldly success. But it's also a prerequisite for continued yogic development. Through increasing self-control, prana is strengthened and begins to do its work internally. The body is rendered fit and further purified. The mind is uplifted and readied for meditation. Regular meditation allows the energy centers to be activated one by one with all their attendant benefits. Eventually, the continual modifications of the dualistic mind are slowly extinguished. Each of these steps is a distinct stage of growth. This is a very gradual path.

In affirming their shared goal, I am not saying these paths are the same, or implying they produce the same results if carried through to completion. Swami Kripalu taught them as different paths that produce different results. What I am saying is the effective practice of both these paths can be informed by the same theory and model of the yogic body. Here are a few points especially pertinent for householder practice.

START WHERE YOU ARE

Before any meaningful action can be taken to activate the evolutionary energy, a practitioner must come to terms with the reality of their current state. Yoga describes the kundalini of most people as being "asleep," where a psychologist might use the term "suppressed." Swami Kripalu describes the mindset that supports its slumber.

Ordinary people come into abundant contact with the Goddess Kundalini as the core aliveness and appetites of their own body-mind, but they fail to recognize her. Caught in the snare of pleasure seeking, she sleeps as they indulge and overburden the senses, which keeps them in bondage. Many are the people who cripple themselves by keeping their energy low, just high enough to function acceptably under ordinary circumstances, and by doing so lose the power to act boldly and creatively.

The first and most important of all yoga practices is establishing the kind of health-enhancing lifestyle taught by SK and detailed in my prior book. Only a person enjoying the virtuous cycle of energy building that results can proceed further on the householder path.

ON THE MAT PRACTICE

Being a householder does not exempt you from the need to get on your mat and cushion.[2] Regular spiritual practice is a critical element in any yogic method of awakening because it provides a safe space where the primal energies are freed from their weighty interpersonal and societal entanglements. Through working directly with the body and breath, these energies can be aroused in a supportive setting that invites them to evolve into their higher expressions. This emphasis on embodied practice is what distinguishes yoga from many other approaches to healing and growth, which clearly point out the need to do this inner work but lack the tools required to accomplish it.

The continual practice of yogic techniques is indispensable for householders and renunciates alike. Householders honor their duties in life and practice up to a limit of two hours per day to maintain good health and partially awaken the evolutionary force. Doing this sadhana, a householder enlivens the subtle body and gradually develops the following worldly powers: personal strength, determination, clear and logical thinking, good memory, creativity, and decisiveness.

The yogic ideal for a householder is to engage in an initial period of focused practice until certain signs appear. Partial awakenings often—but not always—begin in this dynamic fashion. For a period of hours or days, and in some cases longer, a practitioner experiences an upsurge of energy. Accompanying this upsurge may be an elevated mind state and heightened emotional sensitivity. Insights and knowings can come one after another. All sorts of feelings may arise unbidden, and sometimes

[2] Swami Kripalu was clear that some form of regular physical exercise was a critical component of any yogic path. Instead of mandating asana practice, he recognized that many different forms of exercise could be combined with pranayama and meditation on householder path. While he believed the practice of yoga postures offered unique and important benefits, he did not teach that asana practice was indispensable, as was the case with meditation and pranayama.

in inconvenient settings. Sleep may be disrupted by vivid dreams. One or more of the symptoms associated with a strong kundalini awakening as noted in the previous chapter may appear. After instigating a series of inner shifts and outer behavioral changes, this high-energy phase almost always fades out. Afterward, the householder's body-mind and consciousness settles into a new normal conducive to ongoing development.

The value of a partial awakening does not lie in its onset symptoms, but in the lasting gifts it bestows. Foremost among these gifts are a heightened kinesthetic and emotional sensitivity, coupled with increased access to a guiding intuitive intelligence. It is these capacities, if utilized, that allow a person to conduct their lives in purposeful ways that keep the evolutionary force active. The result is an organic process of healing, growth, and empowered action that takes place over the course of a decade or two, and is often likened to the way fruit sets, forms, and ripens on the vine. Swami Kripalu describes the mindset that supports a householder yoga practice delivering on the promise of a partial kundalini awakening.[3]

We all know that when a person is frugal their life becomes more prosperous. Similarly, if you desire to have more energy, you must first ask yourself, "Where does my energy go?" Begin with healthy lifestyle, eating wholesome foods and exercising to maintain alertness in the body and joy in the mind. But all of your resources must be utilized properly to activate the latent energies necessary to awaken spiritually. Discover what yogic practices leave you feeling filled with energy. Where a person over-indulging the senses loses energy, a person practicing brahmacharya (moderation) and yoga becomes a storehouse of energy. When energy awakens, your techniques and routines will come to life. The body will speak its needs. The heart will open to love. The mind will grow increasingly clear and intent on right action. These are signs that you are regaining your full humanity and developing the capacity to evolve to higher states of consciousness. Don't make the mistake of thinking

[3] After significant exposure to Yogi Bhajan and his popular Sikh-based system of kundalini yoga, I believe it's practice, which involves both individual and communal elements, is designed to initiate and sustain the same type of householder kundalini awakening taught by SK and detailed in this chapter outside the context of a residential ashram setting.

mechanical yoga practice alone is the secret. While being trained to race, horses breathe a lot, and sometimes very powerfully, but their kundalini does not awake, and they don't become yogis. To work on the high level to which a true yogi aspires, the practices must be done with the intention to evolve your uniquely human capacities into their divine expressions.

ENERGY MANAGEMENT

People at the ashram often spoke of their efforts to walk the spiritual path in terms of "keeping my energy high." The idea was to keep your vital energy just below the threshold where it became "too much" and made you anxious, manic, or likely to act out in ways that "dumped your energy." A lot was required to walk this path. The ashram recipe combined wholesome and moderate diet, regular exercise, and adequate sleep with daily yoga, breathwork, group chanting, and free-form dancing. The ashram was also a celibate community outside of marriage, with everyone encouraged to practice sexual restraint.

Once a resident got adjusted to living at a higher energy level, there was a natural desire to stay there. Of course, there was also a pull to regress by overeating, over exercising, over working, and all sorts of mostly innocent energy dumping. But by and large, no one had to be compelled to eventually get back on the bandwagon. It just felt better to live from this new place. And every so often, some kind of transformative process would naturally transpire to "bump your energy up" another level. As you can see from this discussion of the ashram lifestyle, SK's householder yoga is not a path of extremes designed to generate a few flashy experiences and afterward boast that "my kundalini is awake." It's a way to awaken the primal force in an understated way and keep it active over many years to foster long term growth and evolution.

When Danna and I moved out of the ashram in 1993, neither of us had a good intellectual grasp of Swami Kripalu's householder teachings on kundalini awakening. Yet, somehow we proceeded to follow them by creating a lifestyle aimed at keeping us what we came to call "soul alive." While our last year in the ashram had been difficult, we had received so much of value from our residency that we consciously strove to "not throw out the baby with the bathwater." We examined each element of the ashram approach, keeping those that still served us, and letting go of those that didn't mesh with our new circumstances. Ever since, we have responded to any individual or shared sense of energetic dullness and stagnation with some shift in our way of living aimed at restoring our sense of soul aliveness. We knew instinctively what some readers may benefit from me clearly stating. Trying to live the full ashram lifestyle outside the context of a supportive yoga community is unrealistic. Fortunately, that's not required. Everyone can find a way to apply these yogic principles to their circumstances and "keep their energy high."

THE ROLE OF CHAKRA MEDITATION

Virtually all of the energy-based paths suitable for householders that I have studied include an approach to meditation in which awareness is focused and then steadily moved up the chakra system. It seems some version of this universally-safe and thus freely available technique is the equivalent of the secret initiations given renunciates simply because of its effectiveness. The mechanism behind all these techniques can be stated in a pithy aphorism. "Where attention goes, energy flows." In other words, if attention is focused on the area of a body in which an energy center is located, it will stimulate and eventually activate that center.

Consistent yogic meditation is the medium through which the gifts of a partial kundalini awakening can be received. Asana or some other form of exercise prepares the body. Conscious breathing activates the nervous system. These are the ways a yogi signals their evolutionary energy that the time has arrived where it can become active. In the moments of mental quiet and depth inner awareness that follow, the awakened energy is invited to ascend the chakras and do its inner work. The goal is simply to sustain a meditation practice that deepens a little each day. Over a period of years, the effects of this can be profound. On the householder path, this mix of asana, pranayama, and chakra-based meditation is the secret energy-raising sauce of the transformative process.

Yoga science teaches that there are seven major chakras, each of which must become active. Upon hearing this, a seeker desires to awaken kundalini and make it move upward, but how can this actually be accomplished? Even without having a guru, a person who follows a regular course of asana, pranayama, and meditation will activate their life energy. This preliminary meditation must proceed to the yogic stage of dharana. The same awakened kundalini that produces spontaneous dhyana in renunciates also results from the regular practice of dharana by householders. It is in this way the dormant kundalini can be partially awakened in the human body and made to activate the chakra system.

This approach to meditation was introduced on pages 22–25. A simple version can be done by breathing into the belly and centering attention at the navel center, then raising and holding attention at the heart center, and then aligning the mind with the pure light of consciousness. For a comprehensive approach, see Appendix 6 and the technique of Divine Descent Meditation.

BE A DISCERNING STUDENT

Swami Kripalu calls renunciation a *path of rapid progress*, but that statement has to be scrutinized. Below, he describes his experience of practicing renunciate yoga after his complete kundalini awakening.

You may be surprised to learn that starting this yoga I firmly believed that I would reach the highest samadhi in six months. As I travelled inside the practice, it looked deeper and deeper still. One year passed, two years passed, ten years passed. Resolute in my decision to travel this path to its completion before undertaking any other activities, I had given up all the distractions of the outside world. Today twenty-seven years have passed with me practicing more than ten hours every day, and yet my sadhana continues.

Looking at his teachings as a whole, this apparent contradiction is resolved. While a complete kundalini awakening and cloistered life allows a renunciate to swiftly progress through the initial stages of yoga, that does not mean they will quickly reach its final destination. My experience suggests that householders may move along their path in a mirror image fashion. Progress starts ever-so-slowly with energy mired in the lower chakras, but as meditation deepens the pace of progress accelerates over time. It's helpful to remember that SK called both of these *paths to the Infinite.* Any subjective sense of forward movement should be mixed with a whole lot of patience.

Some of his teachings suggest *a yogi's energy can be always increasing* and a faithful practitioner can become *a storehouse of energy.* Many of these statements were made in the context of encouraging new students. Ashram life suggests these teachings are not mere hyperbole. People of all ages who take up the practice of yoga often feel like they are building energy and regaining youthfulness. As long-term practitioners, Danna and I see a need to balance SK's new-student encouragement with the reality of the aging process. Now into our sixties and seventies, we're still growing psychologically and spiritually, but no longer have the full get-up-and-go of our youth.

Children and young people appear effervescent because energy is naturally accumulated during these stages of the lifecycle. Conversely, the attractiveness of middle-aged and elderly people declines because energy is lost during these stages. By practicing yoga and conserving energy, a yogi preserves their energetic radiance and forward momentum. This energy-conserving sadhana is genuine because it can be counted upon to sustain yoga's benefits late into life.

What does an active partial kundalini awakening look like in real life? If asked that question, I would point to a person with a vibrant spiritual connection who is able to express the infusion of creative energy that brings in all facets of their life. In his householder teachings, Swami Kripalu downplays the significance of flashy experiences to the point he hardly mentions them. Instead, he emphasizes the more-telling indicators displayed when the initial stirring up of kundalini has passed but its subtle counterpart has remained active long enough to generate noticeable growth:

If done with devotion, the kundalini power can be progressively awakened through regularly performing one or more yogic techniques. In the early stages of this sadhana, an aspirant acquires physical vitality and worldly abilities. In the middle portion, inner darkness and unrest are overcome as mental vacillations are reduced and steadiness is gained. The end stages are entered when real (beyond the senses) knowledge begins to dawn. It could be said that all these are the benefits of yoga sadhana, but in truth they are the gifts of kundalini when awakened gradually through this safe course of practice.

In this broader way of thinking, kundalini is not some sleeping spiritual energy. It's the urge we all feel to actualize our potential. Once that understanding dawns, and a connection is made between the spark of your bodily life force and your capacity to learn and grow, kundalini becomes the indwelling life energy kept vital by a healthy lifestyle that maximizes your energetic aliveness and supports you in accomplishing your aims in life. This is the goal to which the symbology of the yogic body points – meaning the actual outcome sought from enlivening the matrix of the subtle body. When you start cultivating the power of this evolutionary urge in your life and practice, you are walking the path of kundalini yoga that SK taught.

APPLYING THIS CHAPTER IN PRACTICE

As his biography makes clear, Swami Kripalu never strove to awaken the kundalini power. Instead, he got clear on his life purpose and applied the disciplines of yoga to enthusiastically pursue it. Advancing in those disciplines, he created a lifestyle supportive of his bodily health and mental effectiveness, trusting the natural forces to express accordingly. As he moved through the first three aims of life and up Maslow's hierarchy of needs, more of his evolutionary energy woke up (or was unsuppressed) and became available to support his growth. It was all these factors working together that generated his growing potency as a *man of the world* and culminated in the complete kundalini awakening that made him into a great yogi.

It's likely that any reader of this book is already motivated by a strong drive to explore and express their potential. That disposition is what calls people to clean up their lifestyle, find work that aligns with their values, and bring more of their authentic self forward in their communications and relationships. It's also what motivates them to participate in educational workshops, explore different growth paths, and take intensive retreats. If this is true of you, there is nothing you need do other than stay in touch with the felt sense of this drive and answer its call as opportunities present.

Some force flows into us from a realm of mystery to sustain our being and empower our actions. Practicing yoga, it becomes increasingly clear that it makes sense to open ourselves more and more to this mysterious energy and trust it to steer our lives in the right direction.

The yoga sadhanas (systems of practice) by which the kundalini can be aroused in its tolerable form have been prevalent in Indian society for thousands of years. As a result, they present well-established pathways for those possessing both worldly ambitions and spiritual aspirations. Practicing their techniques under the auspices of a competent teacher, the evolutionary force can be aroused to a degree that is not only bearable but beneficial. Individuals fit to tread these paths can be found in substantial numbers and those progressing along them are sure to advance materially and spiritually. To realize these benefits for yourself, find a yogic path that calls to you and earnestly engage yourself in its practice.

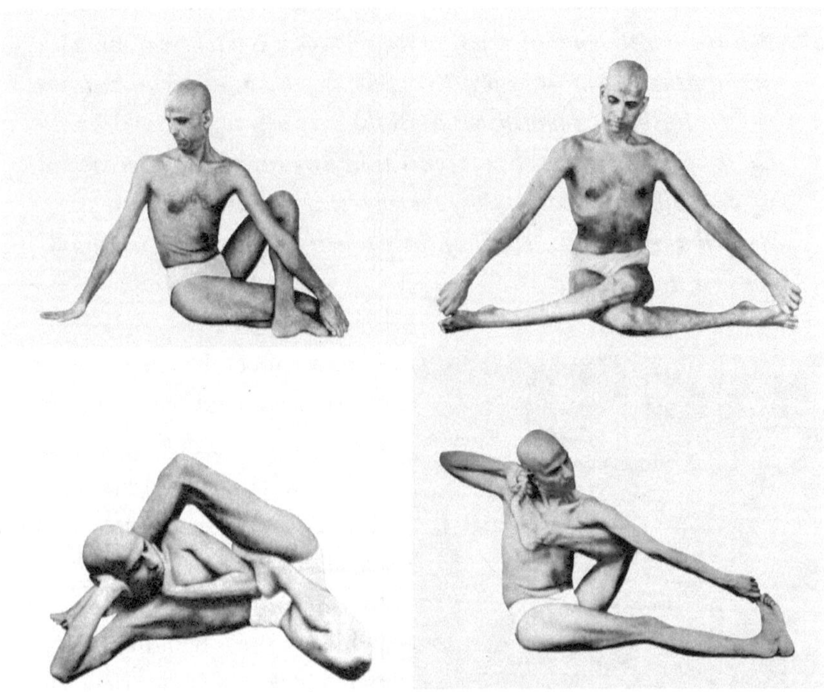

Swami Kripalu practicing yoga postures as illustrated in his book, *Asana and Mudra*. While his ability to assume pretzel-like poses is striking, he also did the simplest of asanas with an elegance and grace.

CHAPTER 7

ASANA AND MUDRA

Postures are the entrance way to yoga, so there is a temptation to see asana as a preliminary practice. But asana has a special characteristic in that it remains vital all the way to samadhi, which is to say the practice of postures is central in any systematic approach to yoga. While the great yogis of the past each favored different poses, they all agreed on the power of their practice and considered asana the first limb of yoga.

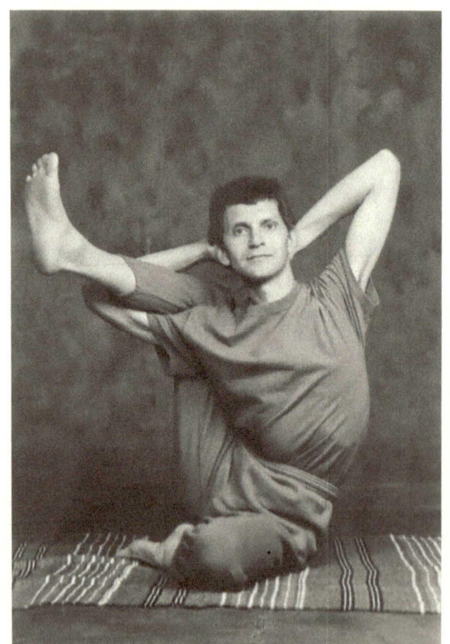

Yoganand practicing Daksina Hasta Catuskonasana in the early years of his ashram residency. This is an easier version of the same SK posture featured on page 7.

I remember the day my good friend Yoganand[1] gave me a bootleg copy of Swami Kripalu's *Asana and Mudra*. We had just finished doing forty-five minutes of pranayama on the carpeted floor of his tiny ashram room. Reaching behind the hanging tapestry that cloaked his doorless closet, he pulled out an unwieldy stack of paper and slid it in my direction. Picking up the title page, I found a rudimentary table of contents that was a long list of yoga postures with Sanskrit names I'd never seen before. Lifting half the stack, I was confronted by a photograph of Swami Kripalu in an

[1] Michael Carroll, whose ashram name was Yoganand.

impossibly difficult pose. Despite this awkward introduction, I felt as if I'd won the lottery.

After carting it home and buying a hefty three-ring binder, I learned this was a partial English translation of a 700-page book written by SK in his native tongue of Gujarati and published in 1967.[2] It opened with an overview of asana fundamentals that included his prescription for posture practice. New students were instructed to learn a balanced sequence of about twenty-five poses that can be done in an hour. Asana practice begins by performing that sequence every morning or at another convenient time. If necessary, it can be divided into two shorter sessions. From there he encouraged students to expand their repertoire so they eventually had several different sequences of twenty-five poses to draw upon. Along with better exercising the body, the ability to alternate between routines prevents boredom. While I welcomed this straightforward guidance, it was clear that some of his Indian readers felt the task of learning fifty or more postures was too difficult.

Thousands of asanas have come my way during my practice of yoga. I originally planned to picture 500 in this completed work. This first edition contains only 277, yet upon its publication people were immediately discouraged and complained, "How and when can we possibly do all these postures?" By eating a few ounces of rice each day, you can consume a mountain of grain in a few years. Taking a daily glass of water, you can empty a reservoir. Similarly, by learning a new pose every day or week, you can eventually master a hundred or more asanas. Physical exercise is as necessary for life as water and food. No one should be upset on seeing the number of asanas illustrated here. All the essential exercises will become easy if you persist in a regular schedule of study and practice.

The overview continued with a set of guidelines for asana students that I immediately began weaving into the fabric of my daily posture

[2] This was in the mid-1980s and a few years before Danna and I became ashram residents. *Asana and Mudra* remained unavailable outside of India until 2019 when an English translation was finished by a team of Charles Berner's students and released by Red Elixir, an imprint of Monkfish Book Publishing, and placed on Amazon.com.

practice. Finding so much of value, I condensed it into a succinct form that spoke to me.

Practiced properly, asana offers equal benefits to men and women, young and old, the ailing and the healthy. Become a student of asana, as the body benefits most when the poses are performed with full understanding. Asanas should be done on an empty stomach. If practicing in the morning, shower and empty the bowels and bladder. If practicing later in the day, wait at least four hours after a heavy meal. If constipation is an issue, practice abdominal poses first to relieve the problem and then continue with other asanas. It is best to wait a half hour after asana practice to allow the body to settle before eating.

Practice in a clean and peaceful environment where there is no strong breeze. Wear loose fitting clothing, and place a thick blanket or mat on a level floor. The ancient teachers of yoga did not have cameras and carved the asanas in rock sculptures that still remain instructive today. If you are learning from a book, study the photograph carefully, read the description closely, and then slowly perform the asana. Start by gently performing the easiest poses with yogic breathing. Gradually increase your endurance by holding the posture longer and breathing more fully. Move on to a new pose only after your gains in strength and flexibility bring this more difficult asana within reach. Notice how long you can comfortably remain in this new asana. Once again, gradually build your endurance by increasing the holding time. The duration of holding and degree of flexibility possible in an asana vary for each individual. Work to your own limit, and do not judge your progress by comparing yourself to others.

While it is good to learn as many postures and variations as possible, a daily practice of about twenty-five is sufficient to maintain health. Start with fifteen minutes and gradually extend your practice time according to your energy and circumstances. Increase the duration at a moderate pace, neither too fast nor too slow, until you are doing a full one-hour routine. After establishing this practice, you may go on to learn fifty or more asanas to give your practice greater variety, but continue to do them in groupings of twenty-five.

Swami Kripalu wrote in a conversational tone that enabled him to easily shift back and forth between topics. Even when offering general guidance, what he had to say held my interest, in part because it felt born from his personal experience.

Follow a schedule of asanas that exercises all regions of the body and avoids excessive use of any particular part. A good sequence stretches and strengthens the head, neck, chest, abdomen, spine, and limbs. While it is customary to learn the classic postures of hatha yoga in a sequence that maintains this balance, most people will find it necessary to start their practice with a grouping of easier asanas.

It takes time to master difficult asanas, and discernment is required to not force the body into them prematurely. Avoid straining the body through over-enthusiastic practice. If you do strain a muscle by forcing an asana, don't be alarmed. Suspend your asana practice and the injury is likely to correct itself within a few days. If the injury does not heal, consult a yoga therapist or doctor before resuming your practice.

No one is truly incapable of asana. If your health is compromised, practice yogic breathing in corpse pose on a regular basis. This is your asana until your condition improves, enabling you to move on to one or two of the simplest poses. Only when these become too easy to bestow any benefit should you try to gain strength and endurance. If by doing this you eventually become vital and vigorous, you will be able to rightly say, "asanas cured my disease."[3]

While doing this work, I kept finding pearls of practical advice that expanded my understanding of asana and are well worth passing on to readers.

[3] SK's guidance included the traditional instruction that women should refrain from asana practice during menstruation. Pregnant women were advised to cease asana practice after the first trimester of pregnancy and wait three months after delivery before resuming their practice. Contemporary thinking has evolved and women practitioners are encouraged to consult more current resources. He also instructed anyone with a health condition to commence asana practice only after getting medical advice.

Some texts and teachers prescribe that headstand be held for three hours. This is not good advice. Ghee is nutritious, but one cannot acquire good health by eating only ghee. However beneficial an asana may be, it should not be done for an excessive period of time. Aspirants should not practice absent this understanding because improper asana practice can bring misery instead of joy.

Many asanas have two expressions in which the position of the right and left sides of the body are reversed. For example, the spinal twist can be performed to either the right or left. There are also complementary asanas, such as when a forward-bend is followed by a backward-bend. Standing asanas are also seen as complementary to asanas performed on the floor. All these classifications are helpful in accomplishing the task of stimulating the entire body while maintaining balance. If you can get an expert to prescribe an asana routine for you, follow their advice rather than insisting on choosing them yourself.

There were also instructions on how to breathe that linked asana to yoga's next stage of pranayama.

Proper breathing is an essential element in the science of yoga and that applies to asana. For example, some poses are entered on an exhalation, others on an inhalation. It is best to follow specific guidance, but some general guidelines can be given. Exhale when bending forward, inhale when bending backward, and momentarily hold the breath when it is necessary to exert energy to lift the body. While performing an asana, one can usually instinctively sense whether inhalation, exhalation, or holding is appropriate. If you are unsure, perform the asana slowly while watching the natural flow of the breath. Often this simple technique is enough to teach you when to inhale, exhale, or hold. Once you are in an asana, continue to breathe in and out normally. It is because performing asana with deep breathing enhances concentration and bestows maximum benefit that I encourage new students to practice yogic breathing for one month before taking up the practice of asana.

The guidelines concluded with a statement that placed asana in the larger context of Swami Kripalu's path of yoga.

> *If you are an aspiring student, engage in a regular schedule of asana practice. If you want to be a true yogi, three other things are needed. First, seek out the guidance of an expert teacher as every asana student needs correction and ongoing guidance to progress into the subsequent limbs of yoga. Secondly, combine asana with a healthy yogic lifestyle. And third, perform your practice while also viewing your work as service to society. Selfless service is the yogic way to strengthen virtues, destroy vices, and build good character. Combining asana with these things will ensure that your practice of yoga leads to an overall success that prepares a spiritually-oriented seeker to meditate with great depth.*

I had learned a lot from the introduction to *Asana and Mudra*, and my spirits were buoyed by its optimistic tone. Turning the page to the posture section, my smooth sailing came to an abrupt halt. It felt like I had entered a foreign world. Almost all of the poses were new to me, and many of those that I'd considered classical postures were nowhere to be found. This was not yoga done in a flowing sequence as taught in the ashram. These were asanas practiced one at a time, and held for prolonged periods, often while retaining the breath and fixating awareness on a particular chakra. While clearly yoga postures, they were practiced in a manner radically different from anything I'd ever encountered. Paging my way through the rest of the book, I closed the binder. What I'd seen was so contrary to the ashram's brand of yoga that I was tempted to simply shelve it. But having run into roadblocks with Swami Kripalu's teachings before, I knew there was more to be learned by persevering in my studies.

After my initial shock wore off, I made a conscious decision to hit the pause button on *Asana and Mudra*. I needed some time and space to review Swami Kripalu's basic teachings. This enabled me to distill his ABCs of asana instruction into a short piece applicable to any posture that I captioned "How to Do a Yoga Posture." Its principles have informed my practice ever since.

All the tools of yoga are meant to steady the mind in a way that brings intense aliveness, one-pointedness, and discerning clarity to your inner experience. While many people practice postures, few know how to perform them in a manner that bestows this steadiness of mind.

Our restless mind can be compared to a pond surrounded by rambunctious children who are continually tossing sand, stones, and pebbles into it. These children are our externalized five senses, whose constant signals keep the surface of our mind disturbed by innumerable thoughts. To make the mind steady, the senses must be calmed so the pond can gradually still.

To steady the mind through asana, you must perform the posture in a way that unites the body, mind, and senses. Start with the breath, breathing smoothly in and out to activate the life energy. Then move into the posture slowly and without hurry. Once the body is properly positioned, become still for a moment, continuing to breathe smoothly in and out. Notice whatever is happening in your feeling body, and allow the awareness of the mind to enter inside and go to the area of strong sensation. As soon as the mind is sent there, the life energy will follow. Allow the mind's awareness, the bodily sensation, and the energy of the breath to harmonize and become steady. As you hold the posture with a flowing breath, watch them unite together in one place. Retain this unity as you slowly release.

When I returned to *Asana and Mudra*, I felt free to simply give it a first read. Instead of using it as a how-to instruction manual, my goal was to learn everything possible to enhance my established posture practice. If I picked up a few new asanas, that would be icing on the cake. This low-key approach worked, and I quickly began finding still more instructional gems that I added to my collection of quotes. I'd heard many yoga teachers cite the Yoga Sutra, which says an asana should be "stable and comfortable" (2.46). While mentioned less often, I knew the next sutra says asana should be done "with the mind focused on the infinite." Swami Kripalu's three-stage process of mastering an asana explained what that meant and provided a road map to get there.

Imagine I was to say to you, "Please stand up." And after standing for a while, suppose I gave you a second instruction, "Now please sit down." To stand and sit, you did not think about the posture you assumed. You gave autonomy to your body, which naturally arranged itself into a comfortable posture. Once a yoga posture is learned, it should be entered and released by means of this same body wisdom. It is best not to think as if a yoga posture should be taken by means of the mind and mental faculty; it is better to allow these postures to occur of their own accord. A person who is truly healthy and at peace will naturally sit and stand in a flow of what could broadly be called yoga postures.

It could be said that every asana is mastered in three stages. In the initial stage, the asana is unsteady. In the middle stage, it is somewhat steady. In the final stage, the asana attains steadiness. The unsteady or steady condition of the body is connected with the quality of the breath and the state of mind at the time the pose is being performed. It is only natural to find a new asana that is taxing to the body difficult. Until the breath moves easily in and out, the muscles will not relax and the mind also struggles. When breathing becomes effortless, the mind can begin to focus inward on sensation (pratyahara) and remaining steady the posture becomes easier. When one-pointed concentration arises (dharana), one reaches the final stage and mastery of the asana is within reach. Through continued practice, a physical and mental capacity develops that makes the asana not seem like hard work. This is the result of correct practice.

While compiling these quotes, I recognized another important theme. Swami Kripalu was quick to recommend that a student round out their posture practice by adding pranayama and meditation to the mix. The below excerpt contains three separate teachings on the relationship of asana, pranayama, and meditation.

Revitalizing the physical body is the first step on the path to spiritual well-being. To make the body healthy, a student should begin to perform the various asanas. This bodily revitalization has an impact on the mind, which in turn grows focused. It is this ability to focus that enables the student to effectively practice the basic forms of meditation. This is why sage Goraksha writes that one should practice meditation only after asana, and sage Patanjali states that it is through asana that the potential powers of the yogi begin to emerge. Once an asana practice sufficient to maintain health has been established, a student should shift their locus of learning to pranayama and the different stages of yogic meditation.

Yogis who shun postures and pranayama (hatha yoga) in favor of practicing meditation (raja yoga) do make spiritual progress. Eventually they discover that they cannot maintain their elevated mental state for long because the lower energy centers are purified and activated only by hatha yoga. It is now known that outspoken yogis of the past who neglected or even laughed at hatha yoga were mistaken. Through their error, we've learned that hatha yoga and raja yoga are complementary practices. Any student seeking to reside in the heights of raja yoga is likely to find that both are necessary, as either one alone proves insufficient.

An ardent seeker of samadhi might think of good health as a trifling attainment and therefore choose not to perform the customary penance of asana practice. But one who has faith in the sages and surrenders to their prescribed path soon experiences how asana makes their meditations more interesting and joyful. This is what gives them the patience to go on practicing and steadily progress to yoga's spiritual attainments. Even when meditation is done on its own, a seeker has to enter an asana (posture) in which they can sit for a long time. In the initial stages of meditation, very few seekers are able to remain still and thus go on restlessly changing postures frequently in order to keep the body comfortable. Asana practice brings steadiness to the body and pranayama brings steadiness to the mind. This is why the yogic scriptures say that it is these different stages of yoga practiced together that reliably bring into reach what is most worth obtaining.

Reaching the end of *Asana and Mudra*, it had become clear to me that SK was teaching asana as a stepping stone to a related but more powerful yogic technique called *mudra*. Yet all my efforts to answer one very basic question not only fell short but failed miserably: What is a mudra? Try and try again, I remained perplexed by this term that I found opaque, yet SK considered seminal enough to feature in the book's title.

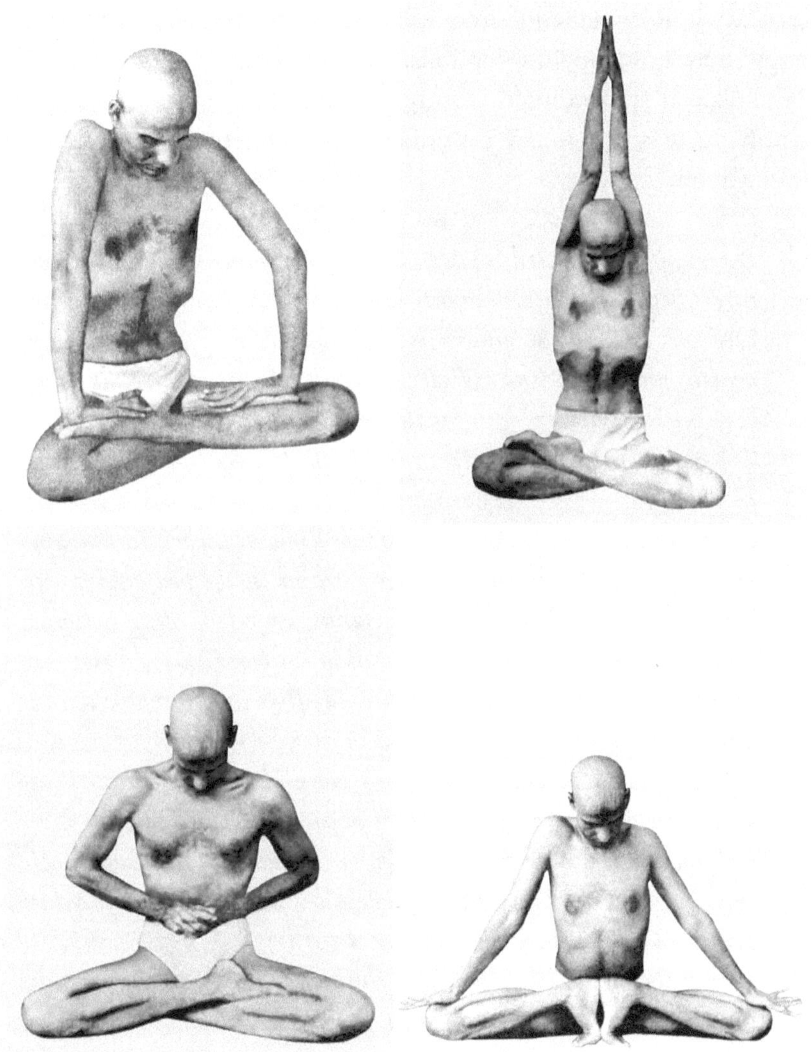

Swami Kripalu practicing yogic mudras as illustrated in his book *Asana and Mudra*.

MUDRA

I can now say that mudra is a hatha yoga technique designed to enliven the subtle body. But back then, I was fumbling in the dark.

In desperation, I looked to his other books and found this glossary entry repeated: *A mudra is a special type of yoga posture with developed pranic activity.* Elsewhere in popular works, I read that a mudra is an "energy seal." Neither of these definitions shed much light on the subject. My inquiry stalled there until a few years later, when I was given a copy of Swami Kripalu's unpublished commentary on the Hatha Yoga Pradipika. It spoke directly to my question, enabling me to compile a clarifying teaching that I captioned "The Difference Between Asana and Mudra."

Externally the mudras appear to be just another grouping of postures. Because of this, students ask, "Please explain the difference between the two." A mudra is a combination of bodily position, breath retention, and subtle internal contractions that come together to create an energy seal. Think of water boiling in a vessel. The steam created can easily throw off the lid. But if the lid is fixed in place, the steam will gain great strength, and a boiler like this can be employed to perform all sorts of difficult labors. In the same way, a yogi uses mudra to activate prana in the body. As prana is made powerful, innumerable asanas, kriyas (healing actions), dharanas (mental fixations), and dhyanas (meditative states) are generated. This is why the scriptures say that innumerable asanas and other yogic rites are concealed in each person's body.

Everyone is familiar with Lotus pose and it can be used to illustrate this difference. Practiced as a posture, Lotus benefits various muscles. If combined with the pranayama of diaphragmatic breathing, it exerts a salutary effect on the vital organs. When practiced with breath retention and the triple lock (tri-bandha), it seals the breath energy in the trunk and becomes a mudra that builds prana and when released powerfully stimulates the gross, subtle, and mental bodies.

Up to this point, what yoga calls *the bandhas* had never made much sense to me. These are internal muscular contractions, often done in the triple combination referenced above, that are said to direct prana into the major energy channels of the subtle body and activate the chakra system. It was now clear to me that the bandhas were the means to engage the desired *energy seal* and produce its pranic potency As I came to understand the theory of mudra, it became apparent that my study was getting ahead of my practice. I was an asana student whose next step was to deepen my understanding and practice of pranayama.

When the difference between asana and mudra is understood, a question arises: "In what order should these techniques be done?" In the Hatha Yoga Pradipika, there are four lessons that cover the subject of yoga from beginning to end. In the first, the postures are described. In the second, pranayama and breath retention. In the third, the mudras. In the fourth, different approaches to meditative absorption (samadhi). It is in this order that the techniques of hatha yoga must be practiced.

BE A DISCERNING STUDENT

The use of postures in India for religious and spiritual purposes dates back at least 2,500 years. In all the early yogic texts, the word asana, which literally means "seat," refers to a relatively small group of sitting postures used to practice breath control and meditation. This explains sage Patanjali's notably brief treatment of asana in the Yoga Sutra, which was written around 200 CE and only specifies that the posture adopted should be "steady and comfortable." More elaborate postures were used by self-mortifying *tapasvins* in their much-older practice of asceticism. A tapasvin might vow to stand on one leg, hold an arm overhead, or hang upside down for days on end to develop the power of their will, or to propitiate a particular god or goddess in an attempt to win divine boons. It is not until the advent of Hatha Yoga around 1,000 CE that texts can be found describing what are often called "cultural poses." These are postures that exercise or stimulate parts of the body or its physiological functions to awaken dormant energies, enhance health, and establish a sense of well-being that aids the spiritual quest. As Hatha Yoga developed, the practice of these cultural poses expanded and the place of asana in yoga moved from a preliminary matter to being an issue of central concern.

The *Hatha Yoga Pradipika* cited by SK is a good example. It was written around 1400 CE and describes sixteen asanas. As Hatha Yoga developed, that number quickly expanded to 84. Hatha Yoga continued to evolve into the 1700s with postures multiplying in number and diversity. By 1800, this phase of indigenous development reached its peak, with complex sequences of postures being taught and the meaning of the word asana broadened to include not only static positions but also dynamic movements. It is during this time that various texts appear describing thousands of postures, including the one cited by SK below. Along with a growing diversity of postures, the goal of their practice also widened to include eradication of disease, maintaining firmness (muscular fitness) of the body, and therapeutic applications to address specific health conditions.[4]

The Gheranda Samhita says there are as many yoga postures as there are living creatures in the universe. Other texts use the number 840,000. Either way, the army of asanas is immense because its role is to activate all the nerve pathways of the gross body and all the nadis of the subtle body. The yogis say that every asana primarily affects one chakra and through its associated nerve plexus, a particular endocrine gland, and region of the body. As the organs in that region receive their proper blood supply and hormonal secretions, many physical ailments and diseases disappear. The yogis firmly believe that all diseases can be destroyed in this way. If a person addicted to drugs, alcohol, or tobacco takes up the practice of asana and slowly builds up to a one-hour limit, they will shed their addiction naturally like a snake shedding its skin.

It was during the 1800s that yoga came into contact with the West and its trending "physical culture movement." Ironically, many of the postures that we most associate with yoga are actually the result of a modernization process that blended Indian notions of asana with British calisthenics and other European forms of exercise. This explains why the asanas taught by Swami Kripalu appeared foreign to me. They are pre-modern and date from the medieval period in which a single asana was practiced and held for a prolonged time, often with breath retention,

[4] For more on this, see *The Roots of Yoga*, page 88.

to activate the process of mudra, which was Hatha Yoga's most important technique.[5]

Yoganand told me that some scholars interpret the definition of a mudra being an "energy seal" in a different light. In pre-modern India, a seal was a wax impression placed on an official document to establish its validity. Such seals were routinely required to travel across boundaries or transport goods from one kingdom to another. Back then, a properly sealed document served the purpose of what today we would call a visa. Seen in this light, receiving instruction in mudra by a competent teacher enabled students to go to inner places barred to them without its imprimatur. Along with mechanically sealing off energies, Yoganand believes the hatha yoga practice of mudra included the ability to access these new vistas in consciousness.

A majority of yoga students are aware that the Yoga Sutra—which is a text to guide the practice of Raja Yoga—depicts yoga as an eight-limbed path consisting of yama, niyama, asana, pranayama, pratyahara, dharana, dhyana and samadhi. Relatively few know that sage Svatmarama's Hatha Yoga Pradipika describes an entirely different approach to yoga as a four-limb path of asana, pranayama, mudra, and samadhi. Learning this distinction explained how Swami Kripalu's practice of asana could look so unfamiliar but still offer me loads of good advice. At the time he wrote and was photographed for *Asana and Mudra*, he was primarily practicing mudras. But having progressed through the lower stage of asana, he could effectively guide the posture practice of students like myself.

APPLYING THIS CHAPTER IN PRACTICE

All of Swami Kripalu's introductory teachings on asana can be applied right away in your practice. Back when I was reading *Asana and Mudra*, I didn't know that a simplified version of his teachings on mudra can be explored in a solidly-established asana practice. Two good poses in which to explore this are Warrior and Bridge. Be aware that this is an intensive form of practice that can roil the emotions. While general instructions are provided below, they should be applied cautiously as this level of practice is not appropriate for everyone.

[5] The hatha yoga mudras are qualitatively different from the hasta mudras or hand gestures practiced as an aid to meditation. See *Dharma Then Moksha*, Chapter 7.

Come into the posture gradually, taking the time required to make any small adjustments needed to feel physically comfortable, while sustaining a flowing breath. When ready, move into your full expression of the posture. Come into stillness, holding the pose like a living statue. In this initial phase of holding, continue to breathe smoothly in and out. After holding the pose for a number of flowing breaths, take in a three-quarters inhalation.[6] Remain steady and still, holding the breath in, allowing the energy activated by the posture to build and grow strong. Let the structure and shape of the posture become a vessel that can contain this energy.

Hold the breath and the posture until you reach the edge of your toleration point, which means that you will move a little outside of your comfort zone, but not beyond your physical or emotional limits and into strain. When the time comes to release the breath, come out of the posture as well. If you are doing Bridge, move into corpse pose. If you are doing Warrior, you might come into an easy lunge with the back knee on the floor. Once again, grow physically still and mentally attentive. Watching the breath rebalance, invite the activated energy to flood the body-mind. Rest until the breath is flowing easily in and out before moving on to the next posture.

It is best to start out performing only a posture or two in this manner around the three-quarters mark of your yoga session. Then end the session with soothing movements and ample time for deep relaxation. Practicing in this manner, you may do fewer postures, but their energetic effect will be more powerful. While this method of doing postures can provide a potent introduction to SK's approach to mudra, the actual mudras are only meant to be applied after steeping yourself in the practice of pranayama, the topic of our next chapter.

Advanced asana practice includes exercises in which the breath is retained either in or out for sustained periods of time. These exercises often include what are called the three yogic locks: mula bhanda (root lock), uddiyana bhanda (abdominal lock), and jalandhara bandha (throat lock). The purpose of these locks is to activate primal energy, concentrate awareness in the spinal column instead of

[6] A three-quarters inhalation allows the lungs to expand as carbon dioxide continues to pour out of the blood stream during holding.

the sensory and motor nerves, and raise the energy into the higher centers. It is necessary to follow expert guidance in these exercises, as otherwise harm can be done. Do not couple asana with the three locks until you have personally studied pranayama with an expert yogi.

CHAPTER 8

THREE TIERS OF PRANAYAMA PRACTICE

Without the practice of pranayama, the full development of a human being is impossible. If you want to rise out of the sea of insignificance by becoming strong and intelligent, if you want to know happiness and prosperity, if you want to gain knowledge of the soul, learn pranayama from an experienced teacher and practice it methodically.

Swami Kripalu was an outspoken proponent of yogic breathing. Studying his talks and writings, his enthusiasm was contagious. It seemed there was so much to know and explore. Long before we moved in as ashram residents, I began to combine my daily practice of postures and meditation with the pranayama techniques he prescribed for aspiring students.

The ancient sages considered pranayama the primary constituent of yoga. Many texts assert that the end goal of yoga (unity consciousness) can be accomplished through pranayama alone. Others emphasize meditation but say that only pranayama can bridle the mind and enable an aspirant to enter its hallowed realms. While yoga embraces many different paths and approaches, pranayama is in some way essential to each of them. It can be said that wherever yoga is being sought, pranayama is being practiced, directly or indirectly. And if an approach rejects pranayama, it ceases to be yoga.

It makes sense that pranayama—the practice of rhythmic, regulated, and purposeful breathing—was central to the yoga taught by SK given the keystone role it played in his own awakening.[1] But studying and practicing alone, it wasn't easy for me to decipher his teachings on pranayama. Just reading in *Asana and Mudra* that there are forty-eight variations of alternate nostril breathing was enough to put my mind on tilt. Applying them safely was also a concern, as he issued frequent warnings on the risk of uninformed or overzealous practice. I leaned heavily on my friend Yoganand, who was recognized as the ashram's foremost pranayama practitioner. The magnitude of the leg-up that Yoganand gave me was monumental. All these decades later, my pranayama practice is still evolving, and I continue to consult him for expert advice.

BREATHING EXERCISES, BREATHWORK, AND YOGIC PRANAYAMA

When I began practicing pranayama in the early 1980s, a cohort of adventurous Westerners were exploring a variety of Eastern traditions and waking up to the power of the breath. Together they birthed a grassroots movement that gained momentum over the next two decades and spawned the ongoing scientific research whose findings make many of today's doctors and psychologists tout the benefits of conscious breathing. In today's mindfulness and wellness marketplace, the word pranayama is rarely used outside of yoga circles. But you're likely to see two terms that help distinguish yogic pranayama from other approaches.

The first is "breathing exercise," which refers to a wide array of breath-based techniques that positively affect the body or nervous system. Some of these exercises focus solely on breathing better or differently. Others combine conscious breathing with physical movements to strengthen the link between body and mind, and often include additional means of amplifying interoception[2] such as inner focusing and visualization. Breathing exercises are usually taught as stand-alone practices done to gain their distinctive benefits. The so-called relaxing breath or physiological sigh is a good example: take a double inhalation through the nose, then slightly purse the lips and breathe out a long, slow audible exhalation through the mouth. When examined closely, this and many other breathing exercises find their origin in yogic pranayama.

[1] For more on SK's awakening, see *Dharma Then Moksha*, Chapter 4.

[2] Interoception is the ability to feel and interpret the sensations and emotions arising within our organism. Conscious breathing is known to improve interoception.

"Breathwork" is a broader term that refers to a systematic approach to working with the breath to produce a targeted set of results. Numerous schools of breathwork have been created in the last half century. Most aim to uplift health by revitalizing the respiratory function through the intelligent application of several different breathing exercises. Others focus on increasing life-hardiness by showing you how to utilize the power of the breath to your advantage. For example, some breathing exercises increase alertness and mental focus, while others remedy stress and facilitate calm. As elite athletes and Navy SEALS know, learning how to skillfully use these tools to remain centered in the midst of challenging circumstances can boost performance and save lives. Still other schools of breathwork seek to catalyze emotional healing, psychological growth, and non-ordinary states of consciousness through specific breathing exercises done intensively to generate transformative experiences.

Even among yoga enthusiasts, the word pranayama is often used to mean breathing exercise. But yogic pranayama is a comprehensive method of working with the breath to increase vitality, uplevel health, facilitate meditation, and spark spiritual awakening. In today's parlance, it is a sophisticated system of breathwork, albeit a time-tested one with ancient roots. Swami Kripalu considered pranayama a *yogic science.*

Today the whole world is becoming attracted to the pranayama of ancient India. The sages of old saw that the life of a human being is an uninterrupted flow of inhalations and exhalations. In practicing as they taught, the process of taking in and expelling the breath is carried out in accord with a scientific method. Unless instructed in the tenets of this science, there can be no correct procedure, and it is a mistake to think otherwise. Pranayama is practiced in an orderly progression. In the beginning, the natural rhythm of breathing in and breathing out is reinvigorated to secure health. In the middle, this natural flow of the breath is elongated and stabilized to produce mental steadiness, and at times suspended to bring about certain beneficial effects. At its end is a state of breathless absorption in which the practitioner becomes established in their true nature as blazing light. This is a concise summary of pranayama science, but to reach its apex you must first grasp its theories, and then practice them as instructed with diligence and faith.

TIERS OF PRACTICE

Hindsight enables me to spotlight the biggest hurdle to my understanding of Swami Kripalu's approach to pranayama. I failed to recognize that he was teaching three distinct tiers of practice, just as the above section reflects. The first tier involves a trio of classic breathing exercises done to revitalize the physical body and facilitate a beginning student's entry into meditation. Swami Kripalu characterized these foundational techniques—*ujjayi pranayama* or the victorious breath, *dirgha pranayama* or the complete breath, and the balancing form of alternate nostril breathing often called *nadi shodhana*—as *useful for everyone.*

Next is a middle-tier in which students explore two more classic techniques—*kapalabhati* or the skull-shining breath, and *anuloma viloma*, the next form of alternate nostril breathing that introduces the practice of breath holding and works to synchronize the different phases of the breath. Each of these techniques employs a different mechanism to increase the flow of life energy through the subtle body to cleanse and open its system of pathways.

The third and final tier introduces another pair of classic pranayamas—*bhastrika* or bellows breathing, and *bhramari* or the buzzing bee breath—that can be practiced alone or together to raise energy to higher levels of expression. In progressing through these three tiers, aspiring students discover which techniques are – and are not – supportive of their physiology and growth paths. In the process, they become able to integrate a rich mix of breathing exercises into their yoga practice.

Swami Kripalu taught that dedicated students moving through these tiers will naturally fall into two groups, which he associated with the householder and renunciate paths. A majority will use the foundational pranayamas to steady the mind and facilitate an awareness-focusing approach to meditation that gradually and partially awakens the kundalini power. The guiding text for these students is the *Yoga Sutra* as clarified by SK's commentary, *Science of Meditation.* A minority will feel called to explore pranayama's advanced techniques, which excite the nervous system and suspend the flow of breath in ways designed to arouse the sleeping kundalini power. SK characterized these pranayamas as *useful for few*, meaning ardent renunciates. If practiced with expert guidance and the requisite intensity, they develop into their own form of energy-raising meditation as taught in the *Hatha Yoga Pradipika* and clarified by SK's commentary, *Revealing the Secret.*

In the following excerpt, he explains how these three tiers of pranayama are meant to be practiced by referencing the four aims of life. In my opinion, this provides a better template to differentiate between students than the broad-brush categories of householders and renunciates. Beginner and intermediate students are to stay squarely focused on the first three aims of life—right living (dharma), material security (artha), and enjoyment (kama)—utilizing the first two tiers of pranayama practice.[3]

Respiration is the driving force behind a human being, as all the bodily systems rely upon its strength, so pranayama naturally plays a central role in yoga. But one must remember the techniques of pranayama are meant to be practiced in accord with the four aims of life. Travelers on the path toward the first three aims of life seek to bring stability to the mental faculty. To do this, they accept the support of diet, posture, and the basic pranayamas (ujjayi and dirgha). Yoga postures are practiced along with walking, running, swimming, strength-building, and other sports or arts (singing and dance) to reinvigorate the cardiovascular system. In practicing pranayama, great attention is paid to regularizing the flow of breath to harmonize all the bodily functions. Progressing along this path, additional techniques of pranayama (alternate nostril breathing and kapalabhati) may be learned to vitalize the body, overcome mental distraction, and ease one's entry into meditation. When used properly, these techniques sharpen concentration and support a meditation practice that generates feelings of deep peace. Through all these disciplines, such yogis gain good health and an alert mind that is clear and creative. They also become capable of

[3] For more on the four aims of life, see *Swami Kripalu's Yoga of Success and Self-Realization*, Chapter 5.

holding a firm intention and acting resolutely in the face of upset. Such steadiness of mind is needed to attain external success and enjoy true fulfillment.

Only accomplished students who had sufficiently satisfied the first three aims of life were ready in Swami Kripalu's mind to shift the critical mass of their focus to the fourth and final aim of life: spiritual awakening and liberation (moksha). This could be pursued through either one of the two yogic pathways he describes below, both of which involve advanced pranayama.

Travelers on the path of accomplishing the fourth aim of life minimize their other disciplines for a time so pranayama can be practiced intensively. Great attention is paid to either slowing the breath to pacify the mental faculty and enter the depths of dhyana (raja yoga meditation), or to suspending the breath to arouse the life energy and cause various kriyas and mudras to occur (hatha yoga meditation). Do not forget that the sadhanas for attaining dharma (success in life) and moksha (spiritual awakening and liberation) are different. It is only this understanding that enables pranayama to be practiced appropriately. This is how the same yogic techniques (healthy living, postures, pranayama, and meditation) can be applied differently by different aspirants to make both human fulfillment and spiritual freedom available.

These two pathways to depth practice are important enough to not only mention but repeat for emphasis. The first is *steadying then slowing the breath to pacify the mental faculty and enter depth meditation*, which is the path of awareness-focusing meditation that emerged from my householder practice. The second is *suspending the breath to arouse the life energy and cause various mudras and kriyas to occur*, which is the path of energy-raising meditation that emerged from Yoganand's renunciate practice.[4] Everything presented about our respective experiences in the remainder of the book is shared to illustrate these two approaches.

[4] After leaving the ashram, Yoganand married and founded a yoga school to teach a form of energy-raising yoga and meditation based on SK's teachings that could be practiced by householders. See pages 123-127 and pranakriya.com.

THREE LEVELS OF PURIFICATION

Swami Kripalu's three tiers of practice arise from the yogic view of pranayama as an expiatory technique, similar to prayer and fasting, employed to burn away a practitioner's past sins and base qualities. In this traditional view, the transformative process is seen as an intensive house cleaning of the entire system called *shuddhi* or purification. Yogic purification is more than cleansing the gross body of impurities that stand in the way of vibrant health. It also aims to remove the subtle impurities said to obstruct energy flow and render the mind unsteady, and even subtler impurities said to obscure the inner light of the soul from shining forth. The traditional terminology comprising this view is presented in the sidebar.

THE PURIFICATION PROCESS AS DESCRIBED BY YOGA

Level	*Sanskrit Terms Defined*	*Contemporary Explanation*
Physical Body	*Bhuta-Shuddhi*: purification of the elements of earth, water and fire considered to be the building blocks of the gross body. Mala: any physical impurity, imbalance, or other obstacle that stands in the way of vibrant physical health.	Physical purification is part of healing. Impurities include a buildup of toxic waste products resulting from poor digestion or other impaired bodily processes, along with unnatural toxins resulting from the ingestion of agricultural and other chemicals. Yoga categorizes the diseases and disorders that result from the compromised function of major body systems as impurities.

Subtle Body	*Sattva* or *Nadi Shuddhi*: purification of the elements of air, ether and awareness said to be the building blocks of the subtle body seen today as the nervous system, mind and emotions. Vikshepa: any energetic, emotional or mental impurity that renders the mind dull, distracted, or agitated. Samskara: subconscious activators of the mind that result from overwhelming, repressed, suppressed, or undigested past experiences. A purified mind is clear, steady, creative, insightful, and non-reactive.	Emotional and mental purification is a complex process generally viewed as psychological healing or growth. Yoga views anything that prevents energy and awareness from flowing freely through the emotional and mental faculties as an impurity. The natural or healthy state is one in which the mind is open to present moment experience and not burdened by residues of the past. Emotional impurities include repressed memories and buried feelings that erect barriers to full feeling. Mental impurities distort reality and include preconceptions, inaccurate belief systems, biased or neurotic thinking, and a variety of defense mechanisms, all of which filter perception, and result in an inability to see clearly.
Causal Body	***Chitta Shuddhi***: purification of the extroverted consciousness that identifies itself as an independent and separate self. Avarana: The subtle obscuration of spiritual ignorance that conceals our true identity as one with Spirit.	Yoga teaches that we have forgotten our true nature as infinite spirit and wrongly identify with the body, mind, and our limited sense of self. False identifications keep us in this state of forgetfulness. All veils separating us from the direct experience of inner and outer reality must be consumed by the fire of purification.

The whole notion of purification may sound like a relic from a bygone era, but it can be explained in contemporary terms. Prior to practicing yoga, many individuals live a sedentary lifestyle coupled with poor eating habits. Consuming too much, exercising too little, and abusing substances causes the body to produce more wastes than it can eliminate. As excess waste products accumulate in the tissues and cells, the body becomes laden with what yoga calls *mala* and alternative health practitioners often refer to as toxins.

The prescription to remedy this situation is yoga practice and healthy lifestyle. Regular exercise and moderate eating allow the body to begin eliminating its toxifying backlog. Asana and yogic breathing enhance this natural process by stimulating respiration, blood circulation, and organ function. Physical impurities that undermine health are flushed from the tissues to enter the blood stream and be eliminated from the system, primarily by the liver and kidneys. Traditional yoga calls this first level of purification *bhuta shuddhi*, the cleansing of the physical body.[5]

Spiritual aspirants are often attracted toward penances that are hard on the body. They unconsciously regard their body as an enemy and fight to suppress it. Such aspirants must ask themselves, "How can self-torture promote inner peace, concentration, and meditation?" True asceticism is not a hatred of the body but a love of purification. For this there is no better penance than pranayama, through which impurities are expeditiously eliminated. As the dross of pure metals like gold and silver is removed by heating them in the fire, so all the dirt and grime polluting the body and mind is burned up by the practice of pranayama. Pranayama is a unique form of austerity because it enables purification to be accomplished without harming the health of the body or diminishing the cheerfulness of mind. But in order for pranayama to be maximally effective, it must be combined with the continued practice of yoga

[5] Chapter Two of the Hatha Yoga Pradipika introduces the practice of pranayama and its opening verse reads: "After a yogi's asana practice becomes steady, that yogi, observing yama/niyama, and taking wholesome and moderate quantities of food, should commence the practice of pranayama according to his guru." This implies that intensive pranayama should not begin until an aspirant has gained a healthy measure of self-discipline and trustworthy source of guidance. Absent those things, the increased energy it makes available is likely to do more harm than good.

postures and diet. Asana, pranayama, and mitahar (moderate eating) are meant to be complementary practices.

Coupling pranayama with meditation allows a parallel process to happen on a psychological level. Anything that prevents energy and awareness from flowing freely through the emotional and mental faculties is viewed by yoga as a subtle impurity. By simultaneously raising energy and relaxing the nervous system, meditative pranayama stimulates these impurities to rise from the unconscious and enter the stream of conscious awareness. On the psychological level, the ability to feel fully and see clearly functions like the liver and kidneys. When unconscious material is held in the light of non-judgmental awareness, it is free to pass through your being, leaving your mind clear and heart open. Traditional yoga calls this second level of purification *sattva or nadi shuddhi*, the cleansing of the subtle body.

Some yoga texts call pranayama the purifying wind because it is capable of completely clearing the channels of the gross and subtle bodies of obstructions. While everyone is continually performing the purifying action of inhaling and exhaling, our overly busy and mentally-distracted lives make the breath chaotic. Pulled in one direction by our desires, and another direction by the demands of others, we are divided. As a result, our minds become agitated. Seeking relief in pleasure, we grow accustomed to overloading the sense organs. Consequently, our system becomes clogged with impurities. Yogis describe this condition by saying "the vital air cannot flow through the nadis." To remedy this condition is a difficult task. This is why instruction is given in the science of pranayama, as through its practice all the accumulated impurities can be dried up.

For most aspirants, obtaining the disease-free state is enough, and this can be accomplished by coupling proper breathing with good diet and regular exercise including yoga postures. Everyone has observed the vital air entering their body, staying for a while, and then going out. In yoga, its entrance is called "filling," its time inside is called "the hold," and its going out is called "emptying." One scientific method of pranayama to clear the channels sufficiently to restore health is to empty all the vital air from the lungs by gently squeezing the abdominal muscles at the end of the outbreath. Next, begin to smoothly fill the lungs from the bottom to the top, taking the time needed to fill all the way to the upper chest. Then hold the vital air inside until expelling it completely once again. Dedicate equal time to this three-fold process of filling, holding, and emptying, as there should be equal importance to each of its three phases.[6]

As the vital air begins to flow more freely, concentration occurs quite easily. Meditation can then be achieved by the proper application of any technique, and the bliss of meditation provides an antidote for the pain of mental dividedness. To succeed in this middle stage of pranayama practice, an aspirant must be faithful and do the hard work of sticking to all of its required disciplines. An aspirant intent on progressing further in yoga should be aware that the clearing of the bodily channels underpinning good health is a prerequisite for the application of pranayama's advanced techniques.

A final level of purification remains that yoga describes as cleansing the extroverted consciousness that habitually looks outward for gratification. Practice at this level aims to remove the most subtle obstacle of spiritual ignorance. Yoga teaches that we have lost touch with the existential joy of our essential self, and as a result wrongly identify with the pleasure-seeking body, mind, and senses. It is this false identification that keeps us in a state of craving and disconnection. Anything separating or veiling us from the direct experience of our true self must be consumed by the fire of purification. What traditional yoga calls *citta shuddhi* or the cleansing of the mental body, contemporary practitioners call spiritual awakening, and it corresponds to Swami Kripalu's third level of purification.

When the body is sluggish and the world is viewed through a thick filter of emotional baggage and mental clutter, it is impossible to see reality clearly and respond with right action. This is why SK taught that

[6] This practice of inhaling, holding, and exhaling for equal measures reflects one of pranayama's basic breath ratios often depicted as 1-1-1. As practice deepens, the ratio gradually shifts to allow more time for holding and exhalation. Practitioners should never breathe in ways that create stress or leave them feeling lightheaded or dizzy, and this technique is no exception.

approaches to growth that do not work to activate prana and purify the body-mind ultimately prove superficial. In the yogic way of thinking, prana is the invisible engine of the transformative process, and pranayama is the direct way to amplify its activity. However, it is important to know the kind of purification brought on by disciplined pranayama practice is not a walk in the park. It almost always entails physical healing crises, periods of emotional catharsis, and the mental pain of confronting unconscious material. That is why he recommended making slow but steady lifestyle changes and deepening your yoga practice at a modest pace.

Once a student asked SK, "I have heard a person needs strong prana to be successful in yoga. How can I develop strong prana?" and he answered:

The prana can be made powerful in many ways. To practice yoga successfully, you must first understand that there are significant differences in the physical condition and mental makeup of every individual. It is because of these differences that yoga offers many tools to increase energy. These tools are not meant to be equally useful to everyone. If someone else uses one tool and find it works for them, that does not mean you will have the same experience. In the past, a guru would see a student's capacities and suggest certain practices. Today it is regrettable that people have to experiment on their own. When doing your practices, you must continually ask, "Am I awake or asleep?" This is because to go forward in your practice you have to pay close attention to your individual experience.

Healthy lifestyle is the primary tool to strengthen prana. After this, the vehicle to go further must be carefully selected. Many people travel best on foot. Others feel comfortable taking a seat on a bus or train. Even though an airplane flies with great speed, there are many who cannot use it. Getting on the plane they feel giddy. If they remain seated for takeoff, they are likely to throw up. Basic pranayamas done to regain the ability to breathe properly and the chanting of harmonizing mantras may be done by anyone without disrupting their bodily rhythms, but the vehicle of advanced pranayama is like boarding an airplane. It swiftly increases the power of prana, but at a speed that causes rapid purification and is hard to stomach.

Most people find it best to grow slowly and steadily. Only you can decide if you are a yogic aspirant fit to travel the path of rapid purification. One guideline applies to everyone desiring to do so. The advanced pranayamas should not be done without the supervision of a capable knower of yoga.

BE A DISCERNING STUDENT

Today, yoga is equated with the practice of bodily postures, but in pre-modern India pranayama was its defining feature. The central role of the breath in religious life was a recurrent theme in the Vedas and Upanishads. A multitude of later texts trace pranayama's evolution from its early ritualistic references into a sophisticated science-like method of spiritual practice. Over a span of millennia, two basic schools of pranayama take shape. The first presents pranayama as an important but preliminary practice that steadies the mind for meditation. The second asserts that pranayama, when done intensively, is alone sufficient to accomplish all the goals of yoga. But even proponents of this second approach admit that it is not an easy way to scale the ladder of yoga.

APPLYING THIS CHAPTER IN PRACTICE

Most yoga practitioners do a few breathing exercises here and there to experience their immediate effects. This makes good sense when taking as little as six flowing breaths can markedly reduce the amount of stress chemicals in the bloodstream and reset the nervous system. Relatively few yogis seek the significant benefits of a systematic pranayama practice. This is in part due to a dearth of instruction from trustworthy teachers like Swami Kripalu, which is why the substantive content that appears in the following chapters and noted Appendices was written.

Today we think of the air we breathe as being composed of oxygen, nitrogen, and carbon dioxide. The ancient yogis believed the breath was also the carrier of prana shakti or the power of aliveness, kriya shakti or the power to act, jnana shakti or the power to know, and prem shakti or the power to love. They saw this breath as originating from chaitanya or pure consciousness, the spiritual source from which all life energy radiates. The molecules of air we inhale and exhale reflect a very ordinary understanding of the breath. It is this esoteric and extraordinary yogic definition of the vital air that should be used in pranayama.

CHAPTER 9

THE FIRST TIER OF PRANAYAMA PRACTICE

Imagine a group of young people go to the circus where they are inspired by the various feats performed. Returning home, each group member begins to practice the act that impressed them the most. It's the same with pranayama. Only by exposing yourself to its different techniques, and observing their capacity to positively shift the direction of your mind and energy, can you determine what is good for you, and what is not good for you.

Swami Kripalu never prescribed a regimented progression of breathing exercises for students to learn and practice. Instead, he emphasized the regular and repeated performance of pranayama's basic techniques, starting with the victorious or sounding breath (*ujjayi*) and the complete breath (*dirgha*) as already discussed. This makes sense given his own training in which SK's guru only taught him a single breathing exercise (*anuloma viloma*) but doing it as instructed caused all the advanced techniques of yoga to spontaneously arise in his practice.

Along with being true to his experience, this style of teaching reflects Swami Kripalu's respect for individual differences. In all areas of yoga, it is incorrect to think that a uniform set of disciplines can meet the needs of people with distinctive temperaments and differing physical capabilities, psychological constitutions, and spiritual inclinations. Absent this understanding, students will strive to conform to some idealized conception of yoga when they would be better off identifying and doing the practices that work well for them. This is especially important in the domain of pranayama, where techniques beneficial for some may prove detrimental for others.[1]

Prana is the energetic link between the living atman and the inert material body. Conscious breathing enlivens this link, which is why pranayama is a vital component in all forms of yoga. Do not think, "There are eight classical pranayamas to learn." It is better to think, "How can I make the link between my soul and body dynamic?" Exploring this way, you may feel called to take refuge in any one of these techniques. Under the influence of this single pranayama, you are likely to find your entire respiratory system becoming more powerful day by day. That growth will bring additional pranayama techniques into reach and make the exploration of them feel natural.

This is not meant to imply that Swami Kripalu failed to discuss the intricacies of pranayama practice, or instruct students in its intermediate and advanced techniques. He did both, but without conveying the impression there was a preordained progression to follow. Yet anyone who traces the arc of his own practice, and compares it with the traditional texts that he studied, will discover there is a template for the practice of pranayama.

As a student struggling to apply SK's mid-tier teachings, I found the strategy of relying solely on my intuitive response to the practices insufficient. I needed a measure of external guidance, which made this framework immensely helpful. Ironically, the best way for me to present it runs counter to his individualistic approach. To paint a picture of what these teachings might look like in practice, this chapter tracks the progress of a hypothetical student through his first tier of pranayama practice. Tiers two and three are addressed in subsequent chapters.

[1] This is yoga's doctrine of *adhikara bheda* or individual differences, which stems from the principle that everyone has a distinctive self-nature or *svabhava* that must be encouraged to come forth and its expression respected. The central role of this doctrine in SK's teachings was introduced on page 73 of *Swami Kripalu's Yoga of Success and Self-Realization.*

A TIER-ONE PRANAYAMA PRACTICE

If you are an on-the-mat yoga practitioner, it's likely that you are already engaged in the first tier of pranayama practice. You may recall from my prior book that Swami Kripalu guided new students to learn a combined version of ujjayi and dirgha pranayamas, which was to be practiced fifteen minutes daily for one month before commencing asana practice. Ujjayi pranayama is literally the *victorious breath.* It's also called *sounding breath* because the glottis is slightly contracted to make a soft sound that is reminiscent of the flow and ebb of waves on the beach. By learning how to make this ujjayi sound and keep it consistent, the breath will flow smoothly in and out of the nostrils. Just as important, a degree of control over the breath is established in ujjayi that carries into all the other pranayamas.

Dirgha pranayama is generally called *three-part breathing* because it stretches and strengthens the breathing muscles of the belly, mid-chest, and upper chest. If done properly, it restores flexibility to the rib cage, which easily becomes rigid as we age. This preliminary period of pranayama practice is meant to jumpstart the process of revitalizing the physical body by restoring your capacity to breathe fully and freely.

Yoga is a science whose tenets can only be only verified by conducting experiments. Sit for fifteen minutes near sunrise and sunset to practice dirgha pranayama. Combine this deep breathing with a wholesome diet. You'll discover that together these practices bring about a marvelous change in body and mind. Appetite and digestion improve. Disease departs as health and self-control return. Awareness increases, worldly capacities gain strength, and spiritual powers awake. Adopt this practice for one month and you will enter asana with your life energy freed up and feeling primed for success.

Swami Kripalu was purposeful in combining these two techniques into a single breathing exercise. A beginning student following this guidance will start asana practice one month later and hit the ground running because it's the steady flow of this sounding breath that is sustained while doing yoga postures. Ujjayi pranayama in the context of asana practice is an even breath, which means the in-breath and out-breath are of equal length and duration. Begin by inhaling and exhaling to a count of three, and gradually lengthen the count to four or more. While sustaining this breath pattern, the *Hatha Yoga Pradipika* teaches that awareness should be fixed on the sensations generated "from the throat to the heart" to keep awareness anchored in the body. That is done by "making a raspy sound that reaches into the chest."

Postures and pranayama are such close companions that the ancient sages made them successive rungs on the ladder of yoga. These are the two means to secure the health of the physical body. Each rung nurtures the other, and only a student who accepts this principle of complementarity will be successful in their practice. It is the same with pranayama and meditation, as only through pranayama can the mental faculty be stabilized.

Ujjayi pranayama is a versatile breathing exercise that can be applied in almost any setting. The Pradipika says it can be done "while walking about (being active), moving the body (asana), or keeping still (in focused breathing practice or while meditating)." In the midst of a dynamic asana sequence, ujjayi is a relatively short and even breath as the abdominal muscles need to be kept firm to safeguard the low back. If sitting erect and still in breathing practice, it's a progressively long breath that involves the abdomen, mid-chest, and upper chest and merges into dirgha pranayama, exactly as Swami Kripalu taught:

After dirgha pranayama has been practiced independently, you need not spend much time on it before doing postures. Taking ten deep three-part breaths at the outset of asana practice should be enough, after which ujjayi pranayama should be continued.

SK recognized that it takes time to establish a consistent breath-based asana practice. Once that task was accomplished, a practitioner was advised to add a short period of sitting meditation. Ideally this follows on the heels of your posture practice, but it also can be done at another time of day. Either way, his counsel on how best to make the move into meditation is to begin your sitting practice with a little time for ujjayi and dirgha pranayamas, utilizing their soothing effects to ease you into the meditative state. Start with a few minutes of ujjayi to smooth out the breath. Gently transition into ten or more full dirgha breaths. Then return to ujjayi, gradually softening the inbreaths and lengthening the outbreaths to calm and introvert the mind.

When should your combined practice of pranayama and meditation begin? The Hatha Yoga Pradipika says that it should start as soon as the posture becomes firm. At this preliminary stage, this should be read to mean that one's asana practice has become firmly established. It is easy to sit down and immediately start meditation, so almost everyone practices in this fashion. But it is more effective to begin with a period of conscious breathing. The yogic scriptures give a lot of importance to pranayama, and my experience is also that pranayama should be done prior to meditation, especially in the early stages of sadhana.

It's tempting to think that we can control our minds by controlling our thoughts. This idea is not entirely false, as it is necessary to apply the will to curb thinking in meditation. But it must be remembered that not all of our thoughts are caused by other thoughts. Many arise from the activity of the senses. This is why the Yoga Bija says that one cannot wean the mind of its thoughts directly. One must first quiet the senses through asana and pranayama, which is the sure way to gain victory over the mind. It's also why the Bhagavad Gita likens the five senses to a team of mischievous horses and says that only pranayama can bridle the horses and enable a yogi to ride peacefully into the region of meditation.

Swami Kripalu believed that it was advantageous for a third pranayama called *nadi shodhana*[2] to eventually replace ujjayi and dirgha breathing

[2] In India, *nadi shodhana* and *anuloma viloma* are different names for one and the same practice. Yoganand told me an interesting story about the origin of nadi shodhana as that term is often used by American yogis. In the early days of the Pennsylvania ashram, the yoga teachers were directed to include anuloma viloma practice in all their classes to reflect the strong emphasis SK placed on the technique. Beginning students found the practice difficult and uncomfortable due to the breath-holding it entails. The yoga teachers responded by substituting a relaxing pause for the hold and the students loved it. Needing a name for this modified practice, they referred to it as nadi shodhana, distinguishing between the two practices in a way that quickly spread. This book follows suit by using the term nadi shodhana to refer to the most

as a means of entering meditation. Nadi shodhana means *energy channel purification* and as taught here it is yoga's simplest form of alternate nostril breathing. Nadi shodhana can be thought of as ujjayi pranayama performed through one nostril, and then the other. In between, there is a relaxing pause that helps you smoothly shift from in-breath to out-breath, and from out-breath to in-breath. Breathing through a single nostril further slows the breath. Smoothly switching from one nostril to the other requires a sustained mental focus that unites the movement of breath with the flow of attention and fosters an experience of inner absorption. But there is also an important balancing effect of breathing through alternating nostrils as explained in Appendix 2.

Alternate nostril breathing is extremely useful for the spiritual seeker desiring to become a depth meditator. The scriptures give lots of importance to this pranayama because the peace or unrest of the mind is very much dependent on the condition of the respiratory system. Yoga likens the right and left nostrils to the strings of a musical instrument. By tuning these strings properly, the meditator's mind will resound with the melody of peace, making even a miserable life full of happiness. Alternate nostril breathing is unique among the advanced pranayamas because its practice is safe. If done properly, it will not harm you in any way.

BE A DISCERNING STUDENT

Anyone consistently practicing yoga's primary techniques—asana, pranayama, and meditation—ceased in Swami Kripalu's mind to be a beginning student. They became a yogic aspirant, as now their practice contains all the elements necessary to take them into the higher stages of yoga. This small shift in nomenclature reflects something significant about the path of yoga. All of us have a body that is sustained by eating and breathing. Some amount of exercise, asana practice, and breathwork may be essential to return the body and respiratory system to a healthy state supportive of depth contemplation.

---

basic variation of alternate nostril breathing that is energy-balancing but not energy-activating because it does not involve any breath retention.

The sluggishness of the body is best overcome by asana. It is with the help of pranayama and meditation that you can successfully continue your journey of yoga. Breathing your way into meditation, the senses are soothed and any remaining thoughts can be easily stilled by the practice of concentration techniques (dharana). In this early stage of sadhana, there is only a need for one of the basic pranayamas (ujjayi, dirgha, or nadi shodhana), because the task of entering meditation can be completed through it. An adept yogi can take a few deep breaths and go directly into meditation. But for now, my advice is to dedicate an ample portion of your meditation time to pranayama.

It's important to underscore what Swami Kripalu means when he states: *there is only a need for one of the basic pranayamas because the task of entering meditation can be completed through it.* In other words, ujjayi breathing can fill the bill, making it the only pranayama you need to learn! Doing the kind of deeper breathing practices described in the next few chapters is not required to grow into your fullness or realize the highest. These more-advanced pranayamas are powerful tools for those who feel called to explore them, but their practice is optional.

APPLYING THIS CHAPTER IN PRACTICE

Swami Kripalu was prescient in saying *the whole world is becoming attracted to the pranayama of ancient India.* Since his death, a tremendous amount of relevant knowledge has been gained through the efforts of pioneering scientists studying the power of conscious breathing. In order to practice pranayama in the informed way that I now know is possible, a student desiring to practice tier one pranayama effectively should familiarize themselves with this growing body of knowledge. To start this learning process, see Appendix 1, *Making Contemporary Sense of Traditional Pranayama.*

As long as the body has life, an individual breathes in and out. Death comes as soon as this flow of breath ceases. This speaks eloquently to the importance of pranayama. Under its influence, the flow of energy through the body and mind becomes greater every day. This is why it is said that the power of pranayama exceeds that of a hundred other exercises combined. But care must be taken to practice it properly, inhaling and exhaling slowly, never straining or forcing, especially when holding the breath. Vital capacity must be gained gradually, or the great power of pranayama may harm the body.

CHAPTER 10

THE SECOND TIER OF PRANAYAMA PRACTICE

Due to unregulated eating, overwork, physical inactivity, and poor sleep, the body's fourteen major energy channels become clogged with impurities. The opinion of yogic science is that the dark and restless condition of the mind results. Accepting this hypothesis, an ardent aspirant begins to practice pranayama (kapalabhati and anuloma viloma) to destroy the impurities blocking these channels. Day by day, the darkness of the mind wanes and its bright condition waxes. The full moon state that results is called nadi shuddhi (energy channel purity), and its light bestows a victory over the shadowy elements of our nature.

It's a mistake to imagine the next two tiers of pranayama practice can be understood through the conceptual lens of physical fitness, nervous system function, glandular secretions, or cutting-edge brain science. They must first be viewed with the same mindset as the yogis who developed pranayama as what Swami Kripalu called a *method of internal purification.* Only after this organizing purpose is recognized and understood in yogic terms can current knowledge be applied to analyze the mechanisms underlying pranayama's efficacy and explore the practical value of its techniques.

While schooled in the worldview of yoga, SK was also a modern thinker. Drawing on his layman's knowledge of health science, he tried to explain how pranayama works to purify the system in a way that bridged this gap.

Yoga says that all diseases are caused by impure blood. More curiously, the condition of the blood is said to render the mind dull and agitated, or steady and sharp, and similarly the emotions as pleasant or distressing. How could this be? Science knows the veins carry deoxygenated and impure blood from the body to the heart. From the heart, it is conveyed by the pulmonary artery to the lungs where carbon dioxide and other gaseous wastes are expelled by exhalation. Liquid and solid wastes are filtered out by the organs and eliminated by the urinary and digestive tracts, or by the skin through the perspiration. The speed at which all these systems operate is determined by the vitality of the respiratory and circulatory systems. In a weak or diseased person, the blood travels slowly and laboriously. In a healthy person practicing asana and pranayama, the bloodstream flows swiftly and easily. Thinking this way, yoga's emphasis on blood purification makes sense.

The purifying workhorse of a second-tier pranayama practice is *anuloma viloma*, the next expression of alternate nostril breathing that builds upon the basic version (nadi shodhana) presented in the last chapter. Anuloma viloma is a breathing exercise with a defining purpose. Various yogic texts designate it as "the technique for purifying the nadis." It is through the diligent practice of anuloma viloma that a yogi seeks to attain the desirable state of *nadi shuddhi* (energy channel purity) in which the primary energy channels of the subtle body have been unblocked and the tissues of the gross body sufficiently purged of wastes to facilitate a free flow of life force through the entire body-mind matrix. By traditional standards, a practitioner who achieves nadi shuddhi arrives at a significant milestone on the path of yoga. Only now are they eligible to engage in advanced pranayama and meditation techniques.

But before delving into the topic of anuloma viloma, it's best to set the stage by examining a preliminary purification technique called *kapalabhati*, which works hand and glove with anuloma viloma to make a second-tier pranayama practice powerful and potent.

SKULL SHINING BREATH

Kapalabhati is a breathing exercise that strengthens the diaphragm along with all the muscles involved in exhaling effectively. Weakness in these muscles undermines health by limiting a person's ability to breathe fully out and therefore fully in. But remedying that bodily deficit is not what motivates most yoga practitioners to take up this practice. Kapalabhati breathing brings an immediate spike in energy that is quickly followed by a feeling of refreshed calm. It's this combination of effects that has drawn yogis to the practice for millennium, a fact reflected in the name the technique was given. *Kapala* means "skull" and *bhati* means "shining," a compound word describing the exhilarating effect of kapalabhati breathing on a practitioner's mental state.

While often taught as a pranayama, kapalabhati is technically one of the *shat kriyas*.[1] In yogic terms, it's a purification technique that powerfully works the diaphragm to offload carbon dioxide from the lungs and eliminate other wastes through the exhalation. It is also credited for cleansing the vital organs by stimulating blood flow throughout the abdominal cavity. Done regularly, it prepares the respiratory system for a smooth transition into the practice of anuloma viloma and eventually the more-intensive bhastrika pranayama.

Skull Shining breath is a rhythmic series of exhalations through the nostrils, accomplished by contracting the abdominal muscles, which lifts the diaphragm. Each exhalation is followed by a passive inhalation through the nostrils, which happens naturally as the abdomen relaxes and the diaphragm descends. The exhalation is short but powerful, being produced by a strong muscular contraction. No effort is made to perform or control the inhalation. As you become established in the practice, you will be able to maintain a smooth rhythm that starts slowly and builds momentum. This can sound a bit like a steam engine that starts up, puffs along a level section of track, and then climbs a steady incline. If done slowly and vigorously, kapalabhati breathing was believed to clean out the "hollows in the head" or sinuses, which is probably how it got its name.

Rapidly expelling and passively filling is known as the skull shining breath. This purifying kriya is the dispeller of disease. Practice of this breath occurs in three stages: ordinary, middle, and highest. When it naturally occurs in the practice of vigorous postures, it is of the ordinary stage. At that time, it expels various elements that

[1] The *shat kriyas* or *six purifying actions* graphically demonstrate the intensity through which the yogis of old pursued their idea of internal hygiene. For a discussion of their role in traditional yoga and the life of ashram residents, see Appendix 4.

molest the body. In the middle stage, skull shining is practiced on its own and the abdomen becomes strong. Here, it stimulates the lungs and organs, amplifying the inner flow of energy to clean out the peripheral channels of the subtle body. In the highest type, the rapid expelling and filling is done like a blacksmith's bellows. Here the skull shining breath has turned into bhastrika pranayama (bellows breathing), which cleans out the central channel and opens the eyebrow energy center. When someone quickly mounts a hill or otherwise vigorously exercises, a natural type of rapid breathing occurs to quicken the circulation and oxygenate the blood. At the time of sexual orgasm, a similar thing occurs. In both of these instances, the flow of energy is directed outward or downward, which keeps the mind externalized. In the yogic practice of skull shining breath, the powerful flow of breath carries the energy upward, which introverts awareness and imbues the mind with a keen focus.

In taking yoga classes from different teachers, I've encountered each of the kapalabhati variations that Swami Kripalu describes. Richard Miller taught a gentle version powered by a rhythmic pulsing of the abdominal muscles that he did for a single five-minute round every morning to stimulate the immune system and avoid coughs and colds. Sikh instructors teach a stronger version called *breath of fire* that is performed in the static positions and physical movements that comprise their yoga sessions. Most ashram teachers stayed true to the slower and more-vigorous expression of kapalabhati taught in the yogic texts. They guided students to sit upright and slightly lift the sternum, which stabilizes the position of the torso. Powerfully contracting the abdominal muscles in this position produces a strong and sharp exhalation. Occasionally a yoga teacher will guide students to breathe in and out so vigorously that the muscles of the chest become involved. Technically speaking, this is no longer kapalabhati breathing but a foray into *bhastrika pranayama*, an altogether different breathing exercise addressed in Chapter 12.

Kapalabhati is a highly-versatile technique. Two or three rounds can be done at the outset of your practice. Take ten long, slow dirgha breaths to warm-up the breathing muscles and prepare the lungs. Then perform 20-50 kapalabhati breaths. Inhale two-thirds of your lung capacity, then hold the breath for 20-30 seconds. Exhale slowly and smoothly, relaxing deeply. Leave ample time between rounds to allow your system to rebalance, waiting until the breath and heart rate to return to normal before repeating. At the end of two or three rounds, move onto postures, relaxation, and meditation.

Kapalabhati can also be practiced in short spurts while holding select postures.[2] Come into the posture and engage ujjayi pranayama to begin the holding process. As you approach the end of your normal holding capacity, perform 10-15 kapalabhati breaths. Then inhale two-thirds of your lung capacity and hold both the posture and the breath for 20-30 seconds. Exhale and release the posture, coming into a comfortable resting position until the breath returns to normal.

For the purposes sought in a tier two pranayama practice, the most important application of kapalabhati breathing is when two or three rounds are done immediately before the practice of alternate nostril breathing. This opens the nostrils, amps up the flow of life force through the nervous system, heightens inner awareness, and lends considerable power to the experience of either nadi shodhana or anuloma viloma.

Always practice kapalabhati breathing on an empty stomach. If you feel light-headed or short of breath, slow down the pace and make sure you are completely relaxing the abdomen after each exhalation, which is the key to a passive inhalation that takes in enough air. If the practice initially feels awkward, know that's normal. It takes some time to strengthen the abdominal muscles and learn how to coordinate your breath with the movement of the diaphragm. If after practicing you continue to feel dizzy, light headed, anxious, or irritable, either decrease the number of exhalations, or the number of rounds, or stop altogether and resume the practice of ujjayi and dirgha breathing.[3]

[2] It's important to note that not all posture are suitable or safe for this practice. For example, kapalabhati breathing can result in dizziness. If done in balancing poses, this creates a risk of fall. In many postures, the ability of the diaphragm to move freely is compromised. The instructional information in this and subsequent chapters is general and meant to round out our discussion of yogic pranayama. Consult a qualified teacher to learn these techniques with the detail required to practice them safely and effectively.

[3] Kapalabhati is an intensive breathing exercise that should not be practiced if you are menstruating, pregnant, have unmedicated high blood pressure, have recently undergone major surgery, or have any other active injury or inflammation in the abdomen or chest. Kapalabhati should not be practiced if you have a head cold or other condition that leaves your head stuffed up. Allow the condition to pass, then resume your practice.

ANULOMA VILOMA

It would be hard to overstate the importance Swami Kripalu placed on the proper and persistent practice of anuloma viloma. As all the ashram residents knew, this was the one breathing exercise that his miracle-working guru had taught him. Practicing it exactly as prescribed is what led to SK's mid-life kundalini awakening. But there was more to his belief in the purifying power of this technique than legend and lore. The following excerpt was taken from a book section he captioned *Anuloma Viloma is the Key to Yoga.*

The Svetasvatara Upanishad states that only a novice yogi whose sins have been removed can continue on to the higher stages of yoga. This should be read to mean that the next step for an asana practitioner exercising increased self-control is to strengthen prana and unblock the nadis. The regular practice of anuloma viloma is the direct way to accomplish this task.

Assume a comfortable sitting posture and close the right nostril with the right thumb. Then slowly and smoothly draw in air through the left nostril. When the inhalation is complete, gently pinch both nostrils and hold the breath. After holding the breath to capacity, exhale slowly and smoothly through the right nostril. When the exhalation is complete, use the same nostril to inhale the air slowly and smoothly. When the inhalation is complete, close both nostrils and once again hold the breath to capacity. Then slowly and smoothly exhale through the left nostril. This is considered one round of anuloma viloma.

While other pranayamas also strengthen prana, anuloma viloma is the best technique for unblocking the nadis because it combines breath retention with directing the flow of breath through alternating nostrils. In this way, it keeps the system balanced and strength can be gained without upsetting the bodily humors. Progress in yoga is made more quickly through this exercise than by any other means.[4]

---

[4] While anuloma viloma is widely considered a safe practice, it does suspend the breath. This can upset the system, and SK recognized elsewhere in his teachings that its practice is not for everyone. To avoid problems, start with nadi shodhana, the

Yoga uses a simple analogy to explain the ability of alternate nostril breathing to clear the pathways of the subtle body. In the same way that you might clean a clogged pipe by flushing water through it one way, and then the other way, breathing deeply through alternating nostrils is said to clear the channels of obstructions. This explains why the technique was named anuloma viloma, which literally means "with the grain and against the grain." Swami Kripalu subscribed to this traditional view.

There are eight traditional pranayamas, but the safest and most beneficial is called anuloma viloma. Its name can be translated to mean "natural direction and then reverse direction." It is because the direction of the flow is constantly reversing that anuloma viloma is prescribed by numerous yogic texts as the best method of purifying the energy channels. While working to clear the subtle body of obstructions, breathing through alternating nostrils keeps the flow of prana through the solar (right) and lunar (left) energy channels equalized. It is in this way that imbalances are avoided and latent illnesses remedied.

Along with channeling the breath through alternating nostrils, anuloma viloma introduces the practice of systematic and rhythmic breath-holding. In anuloma viloma, a practitioner is instructed to inhale and "hold to capacity." There is an important limit placed on the length of the hold, as the next exhalation must be long and smooth. If you have held the breath too long, your exhale will be rough and choppy. Any over-holding will also carry into your next inhalation, which should likewise be long and smooth. By optimizing the length of the hold in this balanced manner, and learning to sustain it round after round, Swami Kripalu believed that anuloma viloma triggers a process of cellular purification.

New life permeates every cell of a yogi who practices pranayama properly. It is natural to want to know how regulated breathing can bring about this result. The cells do hard labor to carry out their functions, and wastes like carbon dioxide, urea, uric acid, various

---

gentler variation introduced on page 102, that does not involve breath holding. Any pranayama that involves breath holding should only be practiced under the direction of a qualified teacher.

salts, and other chemicals are produced. Complications take place if these substances remain in the body instead of being excreted, and many disorders start with malfunction of the excretory system on a cellular level. By the proper practice of holding the breath, the cells are subjected to a tolerable level of stress that compels them to release their buildup of wastes into the bloodstream. Once released, deep breathing helps the lungs and other vital organs to expel these wastes from the body. This cellular purification is only accomplished if correct expelling, filling, and holding of the breath is performed. Once taken in, the breath should be held firmly, but expelling must not be done quickly or jerkily. Correct practice of expelling, filling, and holding can be felt by the yogi as a growing alertness of the mind and aliveness of the body.

Most yoga schools guide their students to practice anuloma viloma with a breath ratio of 1-4-2 to synchronize the phases of the breath. This means that an inbreath taking four counts should be followed by a hold of sixteen and an outbreath of eight. Swami Kripalu was well-aware of this recommended ratio, but he felt it was better for new practitioners to begin the practice with a relaxed pause at the end of inhalation. As respiratory fitness is gained, the length of this pause can be gradually extended, while always remaining comfortable and never forcibly holding the breath. With regular practice, a breath ratio of approximately 1-4-2 will naturally result by virtue of the body's proportions and capacities. Practicing in this way also trains the mind to remain calm in the face of the panicky feeling caused by holding the breath to capacity. The mental fortitude that results is useful in daily life and eventually carried into meditation.

BE A DISCERNING STUDENT

While offering modern explanations, SK continued to look at pranayama in orthodox terms as a form of yogic penance in which the residual toxins generated by improper living are purified out of the system. While his biological theories of how this works are innovative, they are scientifically unproven. He offered them to students as the fruit of his own practice.

It is difficult to ascertain what constitutes the state of nadi shuddhi or "nerve channel purity." The *Hatha Yoga Pradipika* states: "The energy channels of a self-restrained practitioner who does uninterrupted practice of anuloma viloma and builds up to a practice of eighty rounds at each of these four times—early morning, noon, early evening, and midnight—becomes pure within three months." (2.10-11) At the age of thirty-eight, Swami Kripalu engaged in exactly this type of round-the-clock practice. After sustaining it for four months, he had the dramatic energy awakening that shifted the trajectory of his life. Decades later and undoubtedly looking back on that experience, he commented on that verse:

The ancient texts say that a yogi practicing anuloma viloma will become free of impurities and attain the state of nadi shuddhi within three months. But this can happen only if the specified 320 rounds are performed in four sittings divided throughout the day. A renunciate yogi should carry on this practice until the energy channels become clean and certain outward signs are observed. These signs include a light and lustrous body, the absence of disease, the audibility of divine inner sounds, and the occurrence of various kriyas and mudras. Householder yogis intent on purifying the nadis should begin with a practice of 15 minutes and gradually extend their practice to 25 rounds per day, done with full concentration. This practice should be continued for a year-and-a-quarter. After this, they should adopt a particular technique of meditation based upon their liking and practice it faithfully.

As an ashram resident, I was already doing a little kapalabhati and anuloma viloma first thing in the morning to wake up before my pre-dawn hour of solo meditation. At the end of morning yoga, I repeated this pranayama combination with the community before the 6:30 a.m. group meditation. Every day after work ended, Danna and I met in our room to do a half hour of anuloma viloma before going to dinner. Seeing my commitment to pranayama, Yoganand had invited me to join him for an hour of anuloma viloma before lunch. What happened when I accepted his invitation and strung together all these breathing sessions would indeed alter the trajectory of my life, but not in the way I imagined. That story is told in the next chapter.

APPLYING THIS CHAPTER IN PRACTICE

Any reader intent on advancing into the second tier of pranayama practice is advised to read Appendix 2, *Pranayama and the Autonomic Nervous System.*

Meditation may commence without any prior practice of pranayama. But unless a meditator's prana is strong, they will have to spend many years in sitting practice before it begins to extinguish the modifications of mind and open the door to samadhi. It is to speed up this process that the study and practice of pranayama is most useful.

CHAPTER 11

MY FAILED ATTEMPT AT RENUNCIATE PRANAYAMA

The road to liberation is meant for everyone. But there can be no true traveler whose body and mind remain as before they started. We may have accumulated endless impurities in this and other births, but these do not really block our way. The purpose of all spiritual disciplines is to cause impurities amassed in the past to come out. In India, the action of removing these impurities is known as yoga, and a person practicing pranayama to travel this road is called "a burner of impurity."

Swami Kripalu's unedited teachings on top-tier pranayama are hard to interpret. Some are anatomically ambiguous. Others are energetically hard to fathom. In places, the experiences he describes lean heavily in the direction of the other-worldly. This is one reason the wisdom traditions are full of stories, as technical instructions that speak to things beyond a student's range of experience tend to fall on deaf ears. The best way for me to present his top-tier teachings on pranayama in the chapters and appendices that follow is to place them in a context by telling you about a time in my ashram life when I was striving hard to practice them.

When I decided to join Yoganand for an hour of mid-day pranayama in 1992, I was thirty-two and physically active. Three years into our ashram residency, Danna and I had a regular lunch schedule. On Mondays, Wednesdays, and Fridays, I would head out at 11:45 with a band of resident brothers to run, bike, swim, or lift weights before showering and arriving at the dining chapel with just enough time to eat and return to work by 1:30. Danna spent these lunchtimes with a group of sisters with whom she walked and ate. On Tuesdays, Thursdays, and Saturdays,

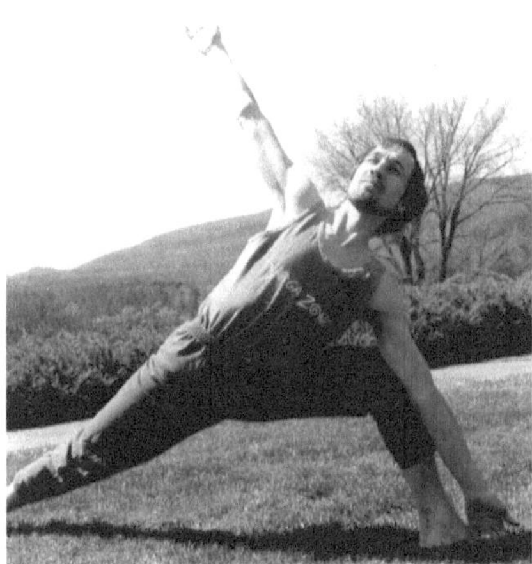
The author in his thirties practicing yoga on the Kripalu Center grounds.

Danna and I would take a brisk three-mile walk and eat together. On Sundays, the two of us would go straight to lunch, which enabled us to spend our precious afternoon off outside and alone, meandering the network of hiking trails that crisscross the Berkshire hills. If we got back to the building before 5:00, I'd go directly to the men's locker room to sauna with Yoganand, who observed a regular schedule of his own.

Doing mid-day pranayama, all the gears of my established schedule ground to a halt. Instead of bursting out the door in my exercise togs to drink in a breath of fresh air and push my body to its limits, I trudged up the stuffy stairwell to Yoganand's tiny third-floor room to engage in what Danna and I started calling "holding my nose." At first, I felt good about the change. I loved exercise and sports, but I'd not come to the ashram to be a jock. In theory, pranayama had the capacity to take the place of all my fitness routines.

Pranayama is the king of all exercises. Under conditions of heightened respiration, the heart, arteries, capillaries, veins, and lungs perform many days labor in only a few hours. As blood circulation increases, basic nutrients are distributed to all the tissues in the body. Waste products accumulating in the cells are eliminated into the veins. Indeed, one can comprehend the significance of all forms of exercise by understanding this process alone. The body parts are moved merely to churn the respiratory process.

I fit right into Yoganand's world. After years of doing shorter pranayama sessions, I easily became absorbed in the tranquilizing flow of anuloma viloma. It occurred to me as an active form of meditation, and I was able to sit for the hour without any difficulty. On most days we were joined by Nijanand, who was one of a dozen renunciate brothers and sisters. This was the first opportunity I'd had to practice with any of them except Yoganand, and I threw myself into it. But a few weeks into this new routine, I started feeling stir crazy.

Along with the loss of outdoor activity, it had quickly become evident that I had to significantly reduce my food consumption. Without the help of vigorous exercise, I couldn't digest anywhere near the amount of food I was used to eating. It was actually worse than that. Anytime I ate even a little too much at breakfast, the experience of noon pranayama went from being a little bit blissful to a whole lot awful. Yoganand ate a single bowl of food each morning, which was mostly yogurt, fiber-less dairy and quickly digesting fruits being the foods traditionally prescribed for intensive pranayama practitioners. For lunch, he filled his one bowl with items from the serving line, and skipped dinner altogether.[1] Before starting pranayama, I was accustomed to filling a plate and bowl at all three meals. If something was particularly good, I didn't hesitate to go back for seconds. As the days passed, I was compelled by intestinal distress to move in Yoganand's dietary direction.

Everything in yoga is done to either suspend or end the modifications of the mind. There are many supportive practices for making progress. Among the most important is mitahar. The word "mitahar" is made up of two separate words. "Ahar" means to eat. "Mit" means "not too much and not too little." For an ardent yogi, mitahar is defined as "eating the precise amount of food required to keep the body alert and efficient." A yogi must accept that it is impossible to stop the modifications of the mind without being careful about diet.

At the two-month point, I found myself really struggling. My body buzzed with frenetic energy, and I was only sleeping a few hours a night. Worse yet, my ability to meditate deeply in the early morning was slipping away. More and more of that once-nurturing hour was spent in a fretful state that I failed to recognize as anxiety. During the day, I felt raw and easily became irritable, a fact my work colleagues pointedly brought to my attention. Looking back, I can say that around-the-clock

[1] These were soup and salad bowls, not the oversized "Buddha bowls" Kripalu Center started offering around 2005. To the best of my knowledge, Yoganand was the only renunciate who practiced the kind of intensive pranayama described in this chapter on a sustained basis.

pranayama was keeping my system stuck on high alert. At the time, I only knew that some type of energetic release was needed for me to sustain this level of breathing practice.

As soon as work ended at 11:45, I started exiting my office to sprint to the end of the East driveway and back, a distance of about a mile. Even running flat out, I was not able to make it to Yoganand's door by our 12:00 start-time. Entering to take my seat on the cushion laid out for me, I'd hear Yoganand's metronome, the steady beat of which made it easier to stay focused on the unbroken flow of inhaling, holding to capacity, and exhaling that constitutes anuloma viloma.[2] Having hurried up three flights of stairs to avoid being late, it took a few minutes for my thumping heart to slow down enough to begin deep breathing. During this lull, something unusual happened. Right after my entry, Yoganand stood up and opened the window wide. This drew my attention, as once Yoganand started pranayama he typically sat still as a statue.

Two weeks passed before a Sunday afternoon arrived when Yoganand and I both ended up in the sauna. Yoganand worked in the ashram's Publications Building, which was located near the end of the East drive. When the morning work period ended, he walked down to his room in the main facility. His ears perked up as I explained why he'd been seeing me running fast in the opposite direction, and then arriving for pranayama late and winded. The exchange that followed was embarrassing back then but priceless in retrospect. I wondered aloud, "Why have you been opening the window wide? The texts say that pranayama is not to be practiced in a drafty place." Yoganand didn't hesitate, "Doing pranayama, my sense of smell is really sensitive, and you stink."

Up to that moment, I'd had no idea that my mad dash down the driveway coupled with all my breathing practice was causing body odor. Yoganand and I were both aware of another verse from the Hatha Yoga Pradipika that says, "The sweat produced from the labor of pranayama should be rubbed into the body." (2.13) We also knew that Swami Kripalu had commented upon this verse: *The sweat of a purified yogi is full of prana and massaged into the body to make it lustrous, but the perspiration of a purifying yogi is full of toxins and should be wiped off with a clean towel*

[2] Quiet music with a slow and unobtrusive beat can serve the same purpose.

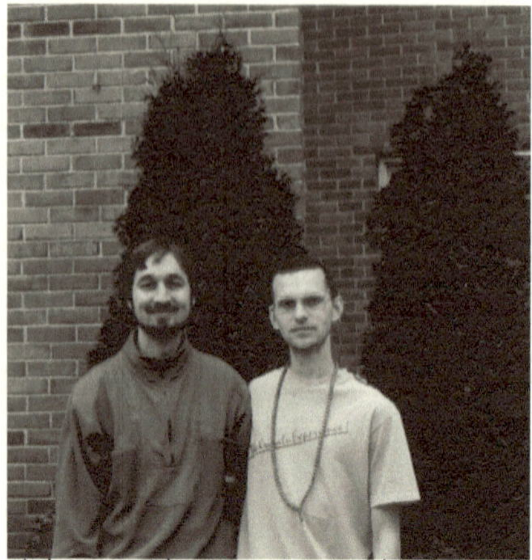
Ashram residents got two weeks of annual family visit time. As an aspiring renunciate, Yoganand spent his doing intensive practice retreats at a small Kripalu-affiliated center in Watertown, New York, with the author chauffeuring him back and forth. This is a picture of them on one of those trips in their pranayama heyday.

after which one should bathe thoroughly. In that moment, there was zero doubt about my status as an impure yogi.

At the time, Yoganand weighed a little over a hundred pounds. He stood out from most of the resident brothers, who were fit and muscular, and the degree of his emaciation was especially apparent in the sauna. It's known that Buddha went through an emaciation before teaching his "middle path" of moderation.

Many renunciate yogic paths still consider a period of extreme asceticism (tapas) like this a necessary step in the purification process. Ignoring Buddha's later teachings, they refer to his actual life story to support this view. My ribs were showing too, but this was nothing new. Even when working out and eating well, I had trouble keeping meat on my bones. But was I really getting purer, or simply disappearing? And mental purity was supposed to bring peacefulness, a measure by which I was failing miserably. At this point, Yoganand had lived in the ashram for a dozen years compared to my three. I poured all this out as if he was my older brother.

Yoganand was kind and understanding. He said the decision to forego vigorous exercise, which Swami Kripalu strongly advocated for non-renunciates, in favor of intensive pranayama was a personal one. Instead of telling me what to do, he asked, "Do you think you are jumping ahead too quickly?" I continued coming to his room for another few days absent the sprinting. But when I announced my decision to return to my athletic lunch breaks, he seemed relieved. Along with being a humorous anecdote from my ashram days, this time in our lives was leading both of us to a fork in the road. But neither Yoganand nor I had any inkling of the changes to come.

The great yogis of the past performed many different practices, but they were all done for the purposes of internal purification. If the purification process is not understood, it can become a hurdle to your growth. The practice of yoga generates tremendous energy, but it also forces impurities to come out into the blood. In the same way the water in a river appears dirty at the time of the monsoon, the blood of a yogic aspirant becomes dirty during rapid purification. Mental irritability and strong sensual desires come forth, and it can even take the form of bodily disease. But beneath these symptoms is the dissolution of the storage bank of impurities. You may feel that you are not progressing, or even regressing, but as long as you continue practicing to the best of your ability that is an illusion. Definite progress is being made, as the amount of purification that normally takes a week can happen in a day, but you are likely not to recognize it. Only as the body is cleansed and the energy channels cleared do we really become disease-free. But great patience is required, as long-lasting purification must be accomplished gradually.

DANNA AND I LEAVE THE ASHRAM

The ashram was a dynamic organism. A few months after my short-lived foray into mid-day pranayama, I was moved into the legal department. There I became embroiled in the guru issues that resulted in Danna's and my difficult choice to leave the ashram a year later in 1993.[3] Hearing the news, Yoganand sought me out. Beyond my friendship with him, he also respected Danna as a yogini. He went out of his way to encourage both of us to rethink our decision. It was an awkward conversation. As a lawyer, I could not be candid about the confidential matters influencing our thinking. In those days, exiting the ashram was considered tantamount to leaving the spiritual path. While neither Danna nor I had any intention of doing that, Yoganand was concerned to see us step outside the supportive monastic structure that meant so much to him.

[3] This story is recounted in Chapter 16 of *Swami Kripalu's Yoga of Success and Self-Realization.*

YOGANAND'S RENUNCIATE SADHANA

Near the time of our departure, Yoganand was included in a group of residents traveling with the guru to India for intensive yoga training at the Kayavarohan temple facility. Excelling there, he returned to become the only resident ever released from the ashram's six-and-a-half-day work schedule to do full-time yoga. He was personally initiated into what Swami Kripalu called *the yogic secrets* without which the renunciate practices done to fully activate the kundalini power cannot begin. After years of preparation, Yoganand quickly left behind the performance of anuloma viloma aimed at nadi shuddhi. Spending all day alone in his room with his door locked, his practice ignited into the high-energy sadhana done by Swami Kripalu in the secluded second half of his life. This yoga is marked by the spontaneous practice of kriyas and mudras, which strongly arouse primal energies.

Where kriyas cleanse and heal, mudras can be thought of as evolutionary actions that bring latent faculties online. Swami Kripalu taught that when the kundalini power of a purified practitioner bursts into full activity, there is an upsurge of energy in the root and sex centers. This catalyzes the first in a chain of mudras. Subsequent mudras allow this energy to coalesce in progressively higher centers, each time building to a climax that eventually brings with it a breakthrough in consciousness. An integral part of this mudra progression is bhastrika pranayama, which occurs spontaneously to raise the energy from root to crown.

Out of innumerable mudras, only a few are given mention in the yogic scriptures. After considerable practice, the kundalini power is awakened. Immediately, bhastrika pranayama and shakti chalana (energy stirring) mudra occurs. This is the inception point from which all the other mudras are generated, so it is noted. The scriptures also praise khechari (moving in the sky) mudra, as with its help the nectar is sipped and samadhi is accomplished. Between these two are all the other mudras and their associated breath holds (kumbhakas), which happen not once or twice, but continually over many years. In yoga's end stages, the indivisibility of its path becomes apparent. It is from this mature perspective in which the whole of yoga is seen as one integrated process that the great sages authored the scriptures. This explains why many texts only describe the first and last of the mudras, as it was not necessary to say more.

In the span of a few months, Yoganand became absorbed in the upward spiral of these renunciate practices. He'd been readying himself to undertake this journey for more than a decade, and fully intended to continue it for the rest of his life.

LIGHTNING STRIKES US ALL

It took the better part of a year for Danna and me to reorient and establish a stable homelife. When Danna landed a professional position in the Salem public library, we bought a fixer-upper house. She resumed the library work she loved. I took a part-time position in a small law firm and began a series of home construction projects. Our return to the workaday world of the Shenandoah Valley of Virginia ushered in a rich but challenging period. Each of us chose to continue our yoga practice and lifestyle, but with greater autonomy and discernment. Together, we strove to "not throw the baby out with the bath water."

Getting up early on weekdays to do a full practice before breakfast, we spent weekend mornings going deeper and then having brunch, feeling our way into a weekly template we still follow. Before too long, I was taking night classes at Radford University, using a master's program in Counseling and Human Development to integrate my ashram experience and put a solid psychological foundation underneath everything I had learned about yoga. At this point, I had no inkling of a householder path to Self-realization. I unquestionably believed the renunciate pranayama done by Yoganand, along with the full-blown kundalini awakening meant to follow in its wake, was the only true path to what Swami Kripalu called *the beyond-mind state.*

Then like a lightning strike from a clear blue sky, the entire Kripalu Center community was rocked by a sex scandal in October 1994. It turned out the financial indiscretions I had encountered in the legal department were puzzle pieces in a larger and more disturbing picture. With zero integration time, all the residents were forced to reconcile their idealized view of the guru with the less-than-perfect man who became all-too obvious. While the wounds were still fresh, the guru made public statements about the number of women involved that proved fallacious. His inability to come clean at a pivotal juncture compounded the situation, injecting incendiary fuel into what quickly became a raging fire. In short order, powerful forces were set in motion that cast out the guru and splintered the once close-knit community into opposing factions.

It would take several years for the ashram to officially disband, but a diaspora began almost immediately that sent residents all over the United States and to several foreign countries. I feared for Yoganand, who I knew was in a precarious position. He stayed secluded in his room for a time, but was eventually compelled to curtail his renunciate sadhana and resume an independent life. Drawing on his work experience in the Publications Department, he found a job operating the printing press of a firm in Albany, New York. Back in Virginia, our new house quickly became a way station for a steady stream of ex-residents moving south.

Someone has asked a question in writing: What is the importance of living in an ashram? In India, people go to the river to wash their clothes. An ashram is like a river where you go to practice yogic lifestyle and cleanse away impurities. In this country, you might say that an ashram is like a laundromat. All of us were raised in conditions where we received favorable and unfavorable impressions. If from early childhood you were exposed to many unfavorable influences, you may need a place that can help free you from harmful patterns. If so, when you become intent on growing, you will naturally run toward an ashram. If you have been fortunate and exposed to many favorable impressions in life, you may feel that you are fine right where you are and have no need to live in an ashram.

Years ago, I was asked a related question: Is it necessary to live in an ashram to practice yoga sadhana? Sadhana requires a safe, peaceful, and uplifting atmosphere. Without this, it is impossible to receive divine inspiration and undergo spiritual experiences. If you can create this surrounding on your own, you can do sadhana anywhere. If not, take up your abode in as ashram every now and then until you can do so. While only a few renunciate yogis will reside in an ashram long-term, every sadhak must grow to love purity enough to want to clean their clothes every day with the washing machine of daily practice.

CHAPTER 12

THE THIRD TIER OF PRANAYAMA PRACTICE

The way in which pranayama is practiced has lower and higher expressions. All the ancient rishis were dedicated yogis, but only a few were practicing pranayama at the highest level. Is this not a surprise? The rishis observed their capacity and never undertook a sadhana beyond their ability. Their system was to steadily progress toward the goal of yoga stage by stage. Modern seekers are intent on finding the highest sadhana but never consider whether they have the capacity to practice it. This approach is not in accord with the teachings of the rishis.

Everything came full circle as I was rehired by Kripalu Center as an attorney in late 1995. Working remotely, I was responsible for all the grunt work required to support a sizeable legal subcommittee of the board and team of outside lawyers charged with resolving over a hundred claims asserted by long-term residents and others harmed by the scandal. By the time that rocky process was wrapping up in early 1998, the organization was teetering on the edge of bankruptcy.

A promising plan had been hatched for the ashram to reinvent itself as a retreat and program center. With staff conflict thwarting the start-up effort, the board precipitously fired an outside CEO with a Harvard MBA who had been brought in a year earlier to turn things around. Needing an immediate replacement, they asked me to serve as president. With so much hanging in the balance, Danna and I felt called to accept, even though that meant selling our newly-renovated home. I was only on the job a few months when the director of the residential volunteer program resigned, enabling me to hire Yoganand to fill the position and resume his rightful role as a yoga teacher. Three years of nonstop work ensued, made possible by Danna's total support.

It was at the tail end of my presidency when my administrative effectiveness was waning that I started writing *Kripalu Yoga: A Guide to Practice On and Off the Mat.* As part of the project, I needed to firm up my teaching status by completing the yoga school's 500-hour training. I was only lacking a single course, Teaching Advanced Pranayama, which was taught by Yoganand. Happy to step away from my desk for a week, it soon became clear that I was lacking more than a credential after my name. I needed to learn two more classic pranayama techniques.

The first was *bhastrika*, a word that means *bellows* and in this context *bellows breathing.* I knew bhastrika pranayama was one of yoga's most powerful techniques. But up to this point, I had reason to ignore its practice. Swami Kripalu taught that bhastrika occurs spontaneously after a strong kundalini awakening. Knowing this, I stuck with my practice of kapalabhati and anuloma viloma, believing that bhastrika practice was premature. Yoganand assured me that I was ready to learn a willful version of the technique that he taught to the group. Digging into SK's writings, I discovered why Yoganand felt this way.

Bhastrika is a pranayama of the last level. In its highest expression, it arises naturally after kundalini awakening and energy-stirring mudra to make the evolutionary force upfacing and activate the chakras. But bhastrika can also be practiced deliberately. When this last-level pranayama is done willfully, it replaces dirgha and anuloma viloma. In their place, 25 rounds of bhastrika may be performed to swiftly rouse the prana prior to asana or meditation practice.

Bhastrika pranayama bestows a unique yogic gift. As long as inhaling and exhaling are performed slowly or through alternating nostrils, prana flows through the two peripheral channels, and the central channel remains blocked. In bhastrika pranayama, inhaling and exhaling take place with great force through both nostrils simultaneously. This causes prana to flow through the channels as one. After bhastrika, the breath can be retained almost effortlessly.

> *It is through this combination of bhastrika and kumbhaka*[1] *(holding the breath after bellows breathing) that the central channel is cleared and the upper energy centers begin to open. Bhastrika is meant to soon be followed by bhramari (buzzing) pranayama, which clears the central channel all the way to the brow chakra.*

As far as I can tell, Swami Kripalu never gave explicit instructions on how to perform bhastrika pranayama. It happened spontaneously in his practice, and that could be seen to explain this hole in his teachings. But it's more likely that he considered bhastrika a potent technique that should not be performed without adequate preparation and supervision. In one place where bhastrika is mentioned, he says *this yogic rite should only be practiced by yogic aspirants of the highest order*, which is why I'd remained a bhastrika virgin for so long. Yoganand had supplemented his study of SK's teachings with an astute reading of verses 2.59-67 of the *Hatha Yoga Pradipika*. Carefully interpreted, these verses provide the instruction needed for regular yoga practitioners like myself to do bhastrika safely.

Kapalabhati breathing and bhastrika pranayama look similar, and both produce a subjective sense of energizing the body. As explained earlier, kapalabhati is a series of active exhalations produced by strongly contracting the abdominal muscles, with the inhalations being entirely passive. In contrast, bhastrika is a series of active inhalations and exhalations. One round of bhastrika consists of a strong inhalation through the nose, followed by an equally strong exhalation out the nose, both of which are powered by a coordinated use of the abdominal muscles, diaphragm, and chest muscles. This bellows-like action produces a rhythmic flow of in-breaths and out breaths with no pauses in-between. There are multiple variations of bhastrika, many of which include movements of the hands and arms that help synchronize the muscular contractions driving the breath. Especially in these movement-assisted variations, it

[1] The word kumbhaka means "to hold." It derives from the Sanskrit *kumbha* or pot. The yogis likened the torso to an alchemical vessel able to contain the *vital air*. When brought to a boil by holding the breath, they believed the vital air rose into the head as a spiritual force. There are two types of kumbhaka. Abhyantara kumbhaka is holding the breath in after inhalation when the lungs are partially or fully filled. Bahya or bahir kumbhaka is holding the breath out after exhalation when the lungs are partially or fully empty.

is important to keep the spine and torso steady while doing bhastrika. Beginning practitioners tend to make this breath rapid and of short duration, when a slower paced and fuller breath taking slightly more time is more powerful.

The vigorous nature of bhastrika pranayama amplifies its effects on the system to a degree that is altogether different from kapalabhati breathing. Yoganand once told me a saying he'd heard in India: "A little bhastrika can help make you a yogi, but too much bhastrika will make you a rogi (crazy person)." In its full expression, each round of bhastrika concludes by holding the breath and applying various *bhandas* (locks). These are subtle muscular contractions that cause the life force to pool in specific areas of the body. SK was outspoken that these intensive breath-holding practices posed real risks. Muscles and joints can be injured by the vigor of their breath-assisted movements. A greater concern is that the body's homeostatic balance and regular rhythms can be upset by the one-two punch of vigorous breathing and prolonged breath holding. Moreover, the mind can be overwhelmed by the unexpected or even explosive surfacing of unconscious material. This is why they should only be practiced under the auspices of an experienced teacher.

An aspirant who has already made substantial progress in purifying the nadis may begin performing twenty-five rounds of bhastrika pranayama. In the same way that a blacksmith impetuously pumps a bellows, the aspirant should move the life energy in the body. In this initial stage of its practice, the vigorous breathing will speed up circulation and sharpen attention. As the practice of bhastrika develops, an aspirant uses various kumbhakas and bandhas to get to know the lower chakras, and then the middle chakras. An aspirant experiencing the upper chakras starts to obtain spiritual wisdom and is truly traveling the path of yoga.

While progress can be made very quickly through this pranayama, an aspirant should expect to confront all the knots (granthis) and obstacles that stand in the way of their growth. That is why it is absolutely necessary that aspirants adopting this powerful pranayama technique be guided by a guru well versed in yoga. All the sages agree on this requirement. A beginning yogi should not bother with kapalabhati or bhastrika pranayama. Concentrate

> *only on learning to breath in a way that the air moves easily in and out of the body without resistance. This is the one starting place for all the pranayamas.*

BHRAMARI PRANAYAMA

After bhastrika, Yoganand taught the group a second pranayama that I had dabbled in but never done methodically. *Bhramari* is named after an Indian insect often likened to the North American bumblebee. To practice this tier-three pranayama, one sits in any comfortable posture and takes a deep breath in. Keeping the mouth closed and lips sealed, the breath is exhaled by making a high-pitched humming sound with the air flowing out the nose. If executed properly, the exhalation is long and smooth, as a nasally but pleasant humming sound is sustained and gradually fades into silence. After learning the basics, we did this buzzing breath for about ten minutes. Everyone experienced its ability to internalize awareness, calm the mind, and generate a mild meditative state. As the program continued, Yoganand led a few rounds to either begin or end sessions. Feeling mentally refreshed, we learned by doing why bhramari pranayama is often taught as a tool for stress relief.

As the program reached its climax, we combined bhastrika and bhramari pranayamas. After a round of bellows breathing, we held the breath in for close to a minute and then exhaled using the humming technique. To aid our inner absorption, we lifted our arms and closed off the ears with the thumbs or heels of the hands, which greatly increases the volume and vibratory impact of the buzzing sound. Yoganand also guided us to lift and slightly roll the tongue back, pressing it against the roof of the mouth, and to visualize the sound emanating from our brow chakra radiating in all directions and reaching into infinity. Three rounds of these two pranayamas done together left the mind incredibly quiet and still.

After the program ended, I wanted to know more about bhramari pranayama and was able to find it discussed in Swami Kripalu's commentary on the Hatha Yoga Pradipika. In contrast to SK's sparse and often cautionary references to bhastrika, his guidance on bhramari is rich and specific, undoubtedly because he considered its practice safe and suitable for everyone.

In order to make bhramari pranayama very clear, I will describe the process of learning it, which begins with the practice of chanting Om.[2] *Inhale through both nostrils and hold the breath in for a time. Then with the mouth wide open, chant one long Om. It is by sustaining this sound that the exhalation takes place. Complete the practice by closing the mouth and inhaling through the nostrils. The in-breath will naturally be quick and deep. Once again, hold the breath in for a time, repeating the process of chanting Om as many times as desired.*

Bhramari pranayama is similar to this method of chanting Om, except the nasally sound of a buzzing bee is made on the exhalation with the mouth closed. This sound is enhanced by a subtle contraction felt in the upper nostrils. It causes the prana to rise into the upper energy centers and stimulate the brain. After bhramari pranayama is done repeatedly, with the sounding exhalation greatly prolonged, the breath will naturally cease to flow in and out for a few moments, transporting the practitioner of this pranayama into meditation.

Continuing my practice of bhramari pranayama after the program, I learned to warm up with a few humming exhalations that generated a pleasant tone resonating in the chest and throat. In later rounds, I found it possible to raise the tone one octave higher to reverberate in the head and at the brow. While bhramari pranayama is generally done to enjoy its gently stimulating and soothing effect, it can lead into profound experiences if practiced after the life energy has been activated by postures or other forms of pranayama.

When the practice of bhramari pranayama matures, the mind becomes transfixed by inner sound. The divine light may be seen, or ecstatic states experienced. Both reveal that the mental faculty is being stabilized. As the mind stills, knowledge from the higher

[2] SK called the practice of chanting Om by its Sanskrit name *pranava*, which means the "infuser of prana."

planes is received. On the way to this knowledge, do not be overly concerned if you sweat, or tremble, or experience powerful emotions, or find tears flowing from your eyes. Trust that the upflowing life energy is stabilizing the mental faculty, which must proceed step-by-step as the tensions accumulated in the nervous system are released. We all know that tension brings misery, and relaxation brings happiness. But the kind of happiness experienced through bhramari pranayama is beyond all the pushes and pulls of duality and rightly called bliss.

A THIRD-TIER EXPRESSION OF ANULOMA VILOMA

After the program, Yoganand told me about an advanced expression of anuloma viloma that Swami Kripalu called *sahita kumbhak*. In this third-tier pranayama, a subtle but critical adjustment is made in the definition of what it means to "hold to capacity." In second-tier anuloma viloma, this phrase means "hold until you feel the urge to release the breath." In third tier sahita kumbhak, the instruction becomes "hold until you are compelled to release the breath."[3]

When alternate nostril breathing is being practiced intensively, this seemingly small change dramatically amplifies its power. In extended sittings, sahita kumbhak will generate a state of inner absorption in which the flow of breath is not only suspended but entirely forgotten. A practitioner who slips into this pranayama-induced swoon will suddenly come back to consciousness and feel they have not taken a breath for a long time. Prolonged holding turns off their time-sense, and sometimes the entirety of their self-awareness. As a result, they are likely to return startled and unable to tell how long they were out.

In places where it was necessary to distinguish this practice from

[3] A second but shorter holding of the breath out after exhalation may also be added, which is performed in the same manner by holding out until you feel compelled to breathe in. The basic breath-retention limits integral to the practice of anuloma viloma stay in place, which means the inhalations and exhalations after holding must remain long and smooth without any gasps or quick movements of the breath. These are important safeguards: see page 112. While internal counting or the use of a metronome may be helpful in learning how to synchronize the breath in tier two anuloma viloma, it is counterproductive in this third-tier sahita kumbhak.

other forms of anuloma viloma, Swami Kripalu drew on the terminology of the Yoga Sutra and Hatha Yoga Pradipika, which define sahita kumbhak as "holding the breath with neither inhalation nor exhalation in mind." In both these texts, sahita kumbhak is one of many steps taken to achieve *kevela khumbak* (the supreme hold), in which the flow of breath comes to a complete standstill and no urge to resume breathing is felt.[4]

When a yogi fills the lungs with air and retains the breath, their heart beat slows. If this pranayama is done repeatedly with the breath being retained for a long time, the yogi may lose consciousness, but this will not last long and they will not be harmed as a result. These swoons (murcha) should not be regarded as enemies. It is not possible to reach the highest samadhi without elevating the mind through them. Yoga distinguishes different levels of murcha in which there may be a blank unconsciousness, or dreams containing thought elements, or thoughtless awareness. The state of swoon in which full awareness remains without the presence of thoughts is a bridge to samadhi.

AN EXPERIENCE OF SAHITA KUMBHAK

Hearing about sahita kumbhak transported me back to an experience I had during our transition out of the ashram in 1993. After four years in the guru-led ashram, Danna and I needed a way to clear our heads of groupthink. In response, we hatched a plan to hike the 500 miles of the Appalachian Trail that follows the spine of the Blue Ridge mountains through Virginia. We'd hoped to start the third week of March, but a 30-inch snowfall closed the trail in the Smokies and many other places. As soon as that had melted, we were eager to hit the trail. Hiking out of the tiny town of Damascus, we felt sure that spring-like weather would

[4] The word *sahita* means "interrupted or broken," a reference to the breath-hold (kumbhak) being interrupted by the bodily need to inhale and exhale, where kevala kumbhak is a synonym for a breathless type of samadhi. Some texts suggest this breathless state can be sustained for up to three hours; others place no limit upon its duration. As his life was ending, Swami Kripalu told his caretakers that it was possible for him to enter a death-like state with no perceptible flow of breath and remain there for hours or even days. See *Dharma Then Moksha*, Chapter 8.

soon follow. Much to our surprise, the cold temperatures and windy conditions continued well into April.

To heft my backpack in the morning and walk through forest scenery all day seemed to me the highest luxury. While I felt full of vim and vigor, Danna was not so impervious to the inclement conditions, which at times bordered on extreme. She managed to keep going by wearing all of the clothes she'd brought in multiple layers, but that made it difficult to be nimble on the rock slides and steep ascents we encountered daily. Seeing her struggling, my energy level rose even higher. During the day, I carried most of our food and gear. At night I slept little, waking up around three o'clock to wrap my sleeping bag around me and do an hour or more of anuloma viloma pranayama, after which I would meditate until the sun came up. In these primitive circumstances, my breathing practice grew very simple. I took a long dirgha-like inbreath through a single nostril. Returning my hand to my lap, I would relax into the holding in the same manner as I might let go into meditation. When a strong need to exhale tugged at my awareness, I lifted my hand to channel an equally long exhalation out the opposite nostril.

One of those days is etched in my memory. The morning began at the foot of a mountain in the Virginia Highlands. By early afternoon, we'd just about reached its summit and were crossing an open bald. The wind was howling, and visibility was terrible. Halfway down the other side, we turned to see that we had been walking through a thick cloud. As dusk fell, we pitched our tent beside a stream and had an early dinner. The wind kept up during the night, blowing loudly enough that it was difficult to tell what kind of precipitation was hitting the tent. Danna was shivering, her sleeplessness made worse by bad menstrual cramps. I was well into my pranayama when something remarkable occurred.

Drawing in a long inhalation, I suspended the breath, just as I'd done so often in my years of pranayama practice. But this time, the dark cold of the tent and everything associated with this world fell away. For a moment there was only a void, but then a crystal-clear story played across the screen of my totally-introverted mind. I saw a wiry brown-skinned man in his late 20s or early 30s. He had a wife and a young daughter. They lived in a mountain valley so high and rugged that it was reminiscent of Nepal or Tibet. Accompanying these initial images was a sense the man I was seeing was me.

I had a small field on the outskirts of the village in which I raised barley. Each spring I would plant, and each fall I would harvest. Like all the men in the village, I did many jobs. But my barley harvest was always sufficient to get my family through the winter. This hard-scrabble, seasonal life made sense to me, and the three of us were happy. Then disaster struck. My wife fell ill and quickly died. It was not proper for a man to raise a young daughter. She was taken away by my wife's relatives. Grief stricken, I could see no reason to plant, no reason to harvest, no reason to do anything. Bereft of all its former meaning, my life no longer made sense, and I simply walked away from it.

For a time, I wandered aimlessly. In the process, I grew to know the mountain passes. Eventually I became a courier who carried payments and other valuables from merchant to merchant. This was risky business, as bandit gangs roamed the mountains paths. To avoid them, I would buy a herd of sheep or goats and blend into the small groups of penniless shepherds common in the region. Sewing whatever was given to me into the padding of a thick fur coat, I didn't hurry my journeys and was never robbed. Reaching my destination, I made it a point to deliver one-hundred percent of whatever I had been carrying to its intended recipient without pilfering anything off the top. As this became known, I was hired by rich merchants and even the kings of small fiefdoms.

The vision ended in a final scene in which I was an old man sitting around a fire with a group of other men. Despite the losses of my youth, I felt content and fulfilled by a second phase of life I'd grown to love. All its lessons could be summed up in two overarching qualities that I'd gained through my experiences: cleverness and honesty. As the story was closing, I wanted to know the man's name. I mentally heard a short guttural word that sounded like "Chen" but remained unclear as to its spelling.

Abruptly back in the tent, I had difficulty re-orienting. Dawn was an hour away, but I needed to get outside and leave Danna sleep. Unzipping the tent door and surrounding fly, I found the world blanketed with an inch of snow. When the sun was finally peaking up, I decided to filter the water we needed for the day ahead. After a difficult night, I wanted

Danna to wake up to a breakfast of hot oatmeal, which required two full quarts. When I heard the sound of the zippers, I looked up to see Danna poke her head out of the tent. Her eyes grew wide as she saw me standing shoeless in a stream, working the handle of the filter pump and holding a Nalgene bottle between my knees. Unable to make sense of the scene, she stammered, "What are you doing?" I was still inhabiting the world of the vision and instantly replied, "Where I come from, there's a saying. If it's flowing, it's warm." After that response, it took quite a while for me to explain myself.

The felt sense of this dream-like vision stayed with me for a few days. It offered a plausible explanation of why I felt so ecstatic wandering in the mountains with my only purpose being to carry a load from here to there. Looking back, I don't interpret this experience as proving reincarnation, although the strong sense of identification that accompanied it is undeniable. But it does illustrate how doing pranayama with extended breath holds can affect a practitioner. Gradually the weather warmed and our hiking gained momentum. Several weeks later while hiking through Shenandoah National Park, Danna stepped out of a phone booth and announced that she had landed the library job that would anchor the next segment of our post-ashram life.

CHARTING THE HOUSEHOLDER PATH TO SAMADHI

After studying SK's life story, I understood how a renunciate yogi uses pranayama to advance toward samadhi. The diligent practice of anuloma viloma and sahita kumbhak produces a state of inner absorption that frees the life energy (prana) from the suppressive control of the mind. This results in the spontaneous performance of asanas and kriyas, which fully awakens the primal power (kundalini), and generate the bodily mudras and extended breath holds the yogic texts say lead to kevala kumbhaka (the breathless state) and samadhi.[5] This was the orthodox interpretation of his path to samadhi adopted by the ashram.

But I had a different question. How does a householder use pranayama to progress toward samadhi? An answer to this non-orthodox

[5] This is a description of the phenomenon and process of *pranotthana* or *prana awakening*. Pranotthana and the practices done by Swami Kripalu before and after he experienced it are detailed in *Dharma Then Moksha*, Chapters 4-8.

question grounded in Swami Kripalu's teachings was harder to formulate. Eventually, I found one cluster of teachings that details the distinctive role pranayama is meant to play on the householder pathway of sitting meditation.

The purification a householder yogi seeks through the practice of pranayama is of three levels: beginning, middle, and complete. When ujjayi pranayama is applied in various postures by a beginning yogi to stabilize the flow of in-breath and out-breath, it is of the first level. At that time, it cleans out the bodily channels, and the health of such a householder yogi is a model to the public. A yogi only becomes acquainted with the subtle body upon entering the middle level of pranayama practice. Here kapalabhati and different forms of alternate nostril breathing are used to cleanse the subtle channels, and the high-mindedness, virtuous disposition, and humanitarian service displayed by such a householder yogi are an inspiration to society.

Beyond this level is the sadhana related to the beyond-mind state (samadhi), which is unrelated to dharma, artha, or kama (the first three aims of life). In this sadhana, there is no thought of profit and loss, social status, or any kind of advantage and disadvantage. It is undertaken solely to become a spiritual person. Householder yogis pursue this through dhyana (sitting meditation), which enables them to concentrate the mind and stabilize the senses. But it must be remembered that flowing between these two (mind and senses) is prana (breath energy), without which there would be no activity of the mind or senses.

In this dhyana sadhana, the pranayama of slowing the pace of inhalation and exhalation is practiced to internalize the mind and senses without any need for lengthy breath retentions. This accomplishes the necessary degree of mental pacification while keeping the mind and life energy at equal strength, which is what awakens the evolutionary force in its partial and tolerable form. After attaining the stage of pratyahara (sense withdrawal) through postures and pranayama, a diligent householder yogi experiences the remaining stages of meditation (dharana, dhyana, and samadhi) one after the other. This is the with-mind sadhana through which a yogi living in society can gradually gain control over all the modifications of the mind and know atman in its original form (Self-realization).

Studying this quote, I grew increasingly confident that I could stay on the path of yoga without necessarily following lock-step in SK's footsteps. And new hints kept surfacing that I was on the right track.

Countless aspirants take up the practice of yoga to find relief from the burning afflictions of life. Some find a refuge in hatha yoga (asana and pranayama) and make it their dwelling place (their sole means to yoga's ultimate goal). Others are drawn to different yoga sanctuaries (schools and approaches) and for them the techniques of hatha yoga (asana and pranayama) provide a firm foundation. Raja Yoga (meditation) is the end stage of all yogic pathways because in it the mind becomes no-mind through samadhi. This is the permanent home sought by all yogis.

BE A DISCERNING STUDENT

Until performing the research that undergirds this book, I had no inkling that the relative efficacy of intensive pranayama and quiescent meditation has long been contested in the yoga tradition. For centuries, this debate was at the root of a doctrinal divide between hatha and raja yoga. The proponents of *hatha* yoga, a word that in this context means *forceful*, asserted that intensive pranayama is required to purify the body and mind. Without it, they argued that efforts at meditation will remain superficial. The *raja yogis* were proponents of *mrdu* yoga, a word that in this context means *gentle* as in *non-forceful*. They retorted that restraining the breath in lengthy kumbhakas is dangerous and unnecessary when safer breathing exercises and easier meditation techniques have proven themselves effective in achieving samadhi.[6] The seventeenth-century

[6] For more on this doctrinal debate, see pages 40-41 of *Roots of Yoga* which cites two raja yoga texts that taken together say: Yoga is said to be of two kinds: hatha (forceful) and mrdu (gentle). Many sages of old died through forceful yoga. Many diseases arise from the inhalation and retention of air, my dear. People die suddenly from them, so one should shun forceful yoga in favor of gentler techniques that pro-

Hatha Yoga Pradipika is famous for bringing these rival schools together. One of its opening verses says: "Instruction is being given in hatha yoga only for the attainment of raja yoga." (2.1) With the general acceptance of this text, the dispute between these schools gradually subsided.

In today's yoga world, hatha and raja yoga are generally seen as two stages of an integrated practice in which postures and pranayama lead smoothly into quiescent meditation. Although hatha yoga is the dominant form of asana practice, few contemporary practitioners employ its intensive pranayama techniques.

APPLYING THIS CHAPTER IN PRACTICE

Any reader intent on exploring the third tier of pranayama practice is advised to read Appendix 3, *Understanding the Advanced Pranayamas.*

Everyone who studies yoga will discover there are many kinds of pranayama. But few realize the advanced pranayamas are their own path and not beneficial for everyone. Perhaps this is why the Jain preceptor Hemachandra Suri exclaimed: "Pranayama is useless. Peace of mind cannot be preserved by it. On the contrary, it generates agitation and the mind becomes depressed." Pranayama techniques are meant to propel a yogi forward and not present obstacles. Hemachandra was a great soul. His statement should make a student of yoga curious. It seems unlikely that Hemachandra was finding fault with the essentials of yogic breathing. Perhaps Hemachandra was exploring an advanced technique but lacking essential guidance? If so, it might have been upsetting his sitting meditation practice.

---

duce the state of yoga in gradual stages. There is no point in spending a long time cultivating the breath, or practicing hundreds of breath retentions that are difficult, painful and can cause disease, or struggling to master all the locks and energy seals, when the ultimate reality can arise immediately by embracing the no-mind state, after which the mighty breath disappears spontaneously.

CHAPTER 13

PRATYAHARA

When a yogi firmly enters the stage of pratyahara, they feel their years of practice are finally yielding results.

Any authoritative source will tell you that pratyahara—the withdrawal of the mind from the activity of the senses—is a pivotal stage of yoga. In Patanjali's eight-limbed schema, it's considered the bridge between the *outer practices* and the *inner practices.* All schools of yoga recognize that it is the capacity of the perceptual senses to not only grow quiet but *turn around to attune inward* that enables the mind to set aside its habitual engagement with the outside world and enter depth meditation.

Despite this universal recognition of pratyahara's importance, there is little guidance on how to practice it. One thing, however, is clear. Pratyahara is not itself a yogic technique. It is a set of mental disciplines applied in other techniques—usually different forms of pranayama, visualization, and meditation—to accentuate their effects. SK's overview of pratyahara includes a basic set of instructions:

In the systematic practice of yoga, control is gradually established over the five senses: sight, hearing, taste, touch, and smell. Because these organs of perception are five in number, it can be said there are five types of pratyahara. But in practice, if steadiness in any one of these senses can be brought about the remaining ones will follow. Pranayama activates the life force and renders the mind introvert, which automatically initiates the process of pratyahara. This is why pratyahara practice is best preceded by several minutes of deep breathing, which prompts the mind to begin to withdraw from the senses.

Everyone knows that visual activity keeps the mind extroverted.

This is why in most forms of meditation the eyes are closed. It also helps if the gaze is raised slightly, as if looking toward the flame-like light of the soul (atma jyoti) that yoga says shines between the eyebrows. This pratyahara of the eyes may be deepened by visualizing different colors either there or in other centers such as blood red, brilliant red, golden yellow, indigo blue, smoky white, pure white, shining clear light, etc.

Once the eyes have grown introverted, it is more difficult to avoid the disturbance of sounds than any of the remaining senses. But if you can get firmly established in the pratyahara of hearing, your meditation posture will become steady and soon the other perceptual organs will grow quiet. In the pratyahara of the ears, you slowly recite a mantra or single phrase of scripture. You can also softly sing a piece of a devotional song or chant in the same manner. In this practice, you must become the speaker and listener at the same time. Enunciate the words clearly, while concentrating completely on the faculty of hearing. Do this by making the right ear very attentive, listening to yourself speak as if you were straining to overhear a secret conversation. Attentiveness is critical in this experiment of speaking and listening to sound, as it is what renders the mind and flow of life force underlying it steady.[1]

Once the theory of pratyahara is understood and a technique is chosen, it must be practiced regularly to bear fruit and begin the progression of stages that define yogic meditation.

The steadiness of mind produced by pratyahara of the eyes and ears may not last long in the initial stages of your meditation practice. But as you become established in these pratyaharas, you will be able to remain steady in longer meditations. Once birthed through the practice of pratyahara, this mental steadiness ensures entry into dharana. Absent this steadiness, dharana and dhyana remain out of reach, making samadhi impossible to attain. Yoga has methods

[1] Pratyahara can also be induced by listening to the spectrum of sounds discernable in your meditation room, starting with those loud or far away such as traffic noise, and ending with those quiet or nearest to you, such as a ticking clock, the movement of breath, and even your heartbeat.

of inducing the state of pratyahara in all the other senses, but these techniques do not need to be learned and willfully mastered. They will naturally occur as you progress in meditation.

In the ashram, the mental disciplines of pratyahara were applied in asana, as reflected in these instructions from an early Kripalu Center publication: "Pratyahara is the withdrawal of the mind from the input coming through the five senses. Pratyahara is cultivated during postures by adopting a passive mental attitude, relaxing the body, performing deep and continuous ujjayi breathing, and moving in an extremely slow and flowing manner. All these elements, when combined, automatically generate the state of pratyahara." At times these instructions were boiled down to a single phase that was to be held firmly in mind while practicing: "Let go of outer distractions and focus your attention inward," and supported by a metaphor used in verse 2:58 of the Bhagavad Gita: "Just as a tortoise withdraws its limbs, so too when a yogi withdraws his senses from the sense objects, his wisdom becomes steady."

These instructions brought depth to my asana practice, and I happily followed them for years to enter a state of inner attentiveness the ashram taught was a stepping stone on the path to samadhi. Then I ran into a statement of Swami Kripalu that said pratyahara could only come into its fullness through coupling it with pranayama, where it served as a bridge to the various stages of meditation:

Success in pratyahara can be achieved only through pranayama. Pratyahara is born in the early stages of asana and breathing practice, but being young it remains weak. When pranayama is at its best, it begins to purify the nadis and pratyahara grows much stronger. As the nadis open, distractions are subdued, the senses become introvert, and pratyahara can be said to have matured. Yet concentration is not complete in this stage. Real stability of mind only arises when pratyahara matures into dharana (fixation). Once it has assumed the form of dharana, the stage of pratyahara vanishes forever and the process of meditation ensues.

Discovering there was more to pratyahara than the asana-assisted version that I knew sent me on a search to learn more, and SK's teachings did not disappoint.

TO PERCEIVE IN THE OPPOSITE DIRECTION

Pratyahara is a compound word that literally means *to draw in the opposite direction.*[2] In our ordinary waking state, the mind is extroverted and busy attending to the constantly-shifting information flowing into it from the outer world through the perceptual senses. In the practice of pratyahara, we begin the process of calming the mind by redirecting our mental awareness to ignore outer distractions and focus within. This complete turn-around of the senses is considered an essential precursor to yogic meditation, which always aims to reconnect us with our core self and energetic source.

There are two clearly identifiable stages of pratyahara. In the first, the mind steps back from the outer activity of the senses and as a result the nervous system grows quiet. Swami Kripalu taught that this stage was best accomplished through the practice of dirgha breathing and the other meditative pranayamas, which act to calm the senses and curb distracted thinking. In stage two, the senses become introvert, which means they start attending to inner stimuli. It is this inner attunement of the sense faculties that generates the introversion of mind required for depth meditation. The practice that SK prescribed for this was *witnessing.*

> *In the wakeful state, we are connected to our surroundings by the sense organs. This makes the mind extrovert, and everything we do is in response to the information received from the senses. During meditation, we want to reverse this situation and receive information from the atman within. To accomplish this, we must temporarily detach our minds from our surroundings by not giving heed to any distracting stimuli. We observe those activities that are spontaneously taking place outside of us as a disinterested witness. This state of witnessing lends neutrality to the mind, quiets the*

[2] Prati means "reverse or opposite direction," and ahar means "drawing off." One of the earliest text references to pratyahara is verse 4.1 of the Katha Upanishad, which says: "An ordinary man naturally perceives outer objects through the opening of the senses. But a brave person of calm mind wishing to know that which does not die closes the eyes and turns sight back on itself to behold the inner Self."

> *senses, and gradually renders them introvert. It is through witnessing that we establish ourselves in pratyahara, the fifth limb of the eight-fold path of yoga.*

It may not be apparent what Swami Kripalu means by taking the stance of a *disinterested witness* in meditation. Imagine that you are going to a doctor's office to receive some important test results. Entering the waiting room, other patients are milling about, and the television is blaring, but you have zero interest in watching the people or the show. Listening for your name to be called, you observe all the other activity as a disinterested witness. This reflects the first stage of pratyahara. To take the analogy a step further, imagine the names of all the other patients are gradually called, leaving you alone. While you are waiting, a show comes on the television that is of great interest to you. Losing yourself in its presentation, you forget entirely about your test results and seeing the doctor. You are startled out of your reverie when a nurse appears to escort you to the examining room. This reflects the second stage of pratyahara in which you become absorbed in the flow of inner experiencing.

HOW DOES IT WORK?

Our capacity for pratyahara is innate. Everyone experiences deep states of sensory introversion in sleep. Swami Kripalu pointed out this connection between slumber, pratyahara, and meditation in a stand-alone sentence: *Yoga is penetrating the sleep states with awareness.*[3] Relatively little is known about the process of waking introversion in terms of psychology and science. Yet anyone who has meditated regularly has seen it in operation. When the mind is introverted, the process of meditation comes naturally, almost effortlessly. When introversion eludes us, meditation can feel a bit like boxing.

[3] This quote stands out from SK's basic teachings on revitilizing sleep and suggests he may have been proficient in the *dream yoga* that plays a prominent role in some Tibetan Buddhist sects. As every lucid dreamer knows, it is possible to have experiences during REM sleep that are informed by the full range of the perceptual senses and closely mirror reality. Some of these dream experiences carry powerful messages arising from the unconscious mind in a symbolic form. I have benefited from lucid dreaming and the science-based teachings of Stephen LaBerge, PhD, along with Robert Waggoner's practical instruction. For a contemporary approach to the nocturnal practices of Vajrayana Buddhism, see the work of Andrew Holoceck.

Traditional yoga explains the mechanism of pratyahara in terms of the subtle body, through which the spiritual energy of atman is said to animate our being. In this yogic way of thinking, it is a strong and steady flow of this vitalizing energy through the network of the nadis and into the body-mind that underlies good health and mental acuity. But the subtle body has a secondary purpose that often goes unmentioned. Out of the 350,000 channels said to comprise the entirety of the subtle body, only one of them flows all the way back to our spiritual source. A yogi undertakes the inner journey of Self-realization by opening this central channel wide through pranayama practice, and then reversing its flow by pratyahara and introspective meditation.

There is a hollow nadi in the spinal cord that emerges from the brain and runs down the vertebral column to the tip of the coccyx. In yoga this is called the sushumna nadi. When this central channel opens and life energy begins to ascend the spine, the lesser nadis and sense organs become actionless of their own accord. The Yogis call this state pratyahara, the quieting of the senses. There is no other way to attain the vision of yoga except by traversing this path of pratyahara because with other methods the senses are not sublimated and the mind does not become immune to distraction.

This explains why so many techniques of yogic meditation focus attention on the energy centers starting with the lowest chakra at the base of the spine and proceeding sequentially to the uppermost chakra at the crown of the head.[4] The idea underlying these practices is that the spiritual energy that normally flows down-and-out through the nadis of the subtle body can be redirected to flow inward from all the peripheral nerves to enter the spine via their regional chakra and then raised up to the crown where the subtle body connects with the spiritual source.

The sushumna nadi is also called the Brahman nadi or channel to the Absolute. Where all the other nadis pass through the peripheral

[4] Two good examples are Kriya Yoga as taught by Swami Paramahansa Yogananda, and the practice of Superconscious Meditation as taught by Swami Rama of the Himalayan Institute. See also the technique of Divine Descent Meditation in Appendix 6.

regions of the body, only the sushumna nadi lies in the spinal column and it alone pierces the chakras. The task of making the life energy enter the spine and mount to the brain is difficult. A yogi must be content to perform the correct practice of pranayama and pratyahara for some time. When all the peripheral channels unite and begin to flow as one, it seems as if a fresh channel is born from them. This is the opening of the sushumna nadi. When the life force starts flowing through it in the direction of the spiritual source, the body immediately becomes motionless, awareness is internalized, and the mind grows deeply absorbed.

Yoganand told me that there are two different yogic models of how the central channel opens. In the first, all the lesser channels close, diverting the energy into the central channel, which opens to receive its flow. In the second model, the flow of life energy through all the channels is unblocked and equalized, which causes them to lose their individuality. Merging into a single flow, they are experienced as one channel flowing back to source. Swami Kripalu references each of these models in the above two quotes. Regardless of how it may be produced, this internal opening is accompanied by a depth state of consciousness notably free of egocentric concerns and mental filtering.

AN EXPERIENCE OF PRATYAHARA

In spring 2022, I was lying on a surgical gurney at the Duke University Medical Center, clad in a hospital gown with an IV in my arm. With all my pre-op tasks completed, Danna had just pushed the curtain of my cubicle aside to keep me company when my surgeon appeared in his scrubs. The marked uneasiness in his voice led Danna and I to make eye contact. He quickly got to the point. The relatively simple procedure I had been told would repair my broken artificial ankle would not work. A much more extensive surgery was required, one that involved fracturing and repositioning my tibia.

This was more than bad health news. A year earlier, my insurance company had denied coverage for anything but an ankle fusion. I had come to Duke as my last resort to keep the ability to walk normally, and we were paying for everything out-of-pocket. To make matters worse,

I'd already had one surgery at Duke the previous fall, but the implant installed had unexpectedly failed, leaving me hobbled with a bulging ankle that was completely unable to bear weight. The first surgery had drained our cash reserves. This second one was a much bigger financial threat. My surgeon ended his explanation saying, "I'm a clinician and don't know what this will do to the costs of the procedure. But if you're going ahead with this, I have to get you right in."

Danna and I locked eyes a second time. The fact was that we had no other options. I signed the consent form. Danna was immediately escorted to the waiting room, and the anesthesiologist entered to give me a mild sedative as a first step in administering a fentanyl nerve block. When both of those things were done, I was left alone in the curtained cubicle, which was open to a wide and active corridor. To divert my attention from all the hospital noise, I started dirgha pranayama. By taking long wave-like breaths, filling my lungs from bottom to top, then emptying them from top to bottom, and allowing one breath to flow directly into the next, I was able to calm myself down. Gradually all the surrounding noise seemed to recede into the background.

About an hour passed when my pre-op nurse returned to tell me they had run into a problem. Too many people were coming out of surgery at the same time, which had created a bottleneck. I was next in line, but it would be some time before an operating room could be readied. I continued doing pranayama and discovered that my vital signs had slowed enough for me to trigger the nurse's alarm by simply pausing my breath for a few seconds at the end of the inhale. I hovered around that spot, just above the alarm's trigger point, for another hour or so, feeling relaxed and present.

When I was finally wheeled into the operating room, I was able to greet my surgical team and thank them in advance for taking care of me. Their stunned silence instantly let me know that I was supposed to be knocked out, and the anesthesiologist was quickly at my side. Going under general anesthesia, the outside world fell away. But surprisingly I remained awake and aware, merged in a luminous field of lovely light, shining like a beacon in a vast and peaceful expanse, completely free of any individual identity. Just as Swami Kripalu taught, all the pranayama I had done was allowing me to penetrate this chemically-induced sleep state with awareness. But I wasn't just seeing this scene as a spectator.

I was this grand expanse—and knew that with a certainty impervious to doubt—because it was not only a field of light but also a network of consciousness that could equally be described as an ocean of love. In retrospect, I can say that no one in this state would choose to leave it. It was permeated by a blissful joyousness that would prevent any such thought from ever arising. The experience was timeless, but I was later told the surgery took about an hour.

In the recovery room, I was able to watch as the layers of my being came back on line one by one. The first thing I became aware of was a subtle and expansive sense of being. There was very little identity attached to this layer, just a hint of differentiation from the larger field. Next came a layer recognizable as an individuated mind, but one so still and steady that it seemed perfectly reflective and mirror-like. Pervading this mind was an overflowing feeling of contentment and well-being.

A next layer slowly took shape as I started to sense my body with a second and more-familiar layer of mind linked to it. The process was intriguing, as I felt and psychically "saw" different regions of my nervous system come online, and eventually join together. At this point my five senses still remained completely silent, isolating me from the tumult of the outside world. Only as my perceptual senses started operating again did I start to regain my normal egocentric identity. The first to return was hearing. Aware of sounds, I was able to detect movement all around me and remembered that I was in a hospital. Light sensitivity and sight soon followed, and my thoughts turned to Danna, the outcome of the surgery, and soon after that the unknown financial implications surrounding it. But even in the face of those thoughts, the overarching feeling of deep well-being remained.

When the recovery nurse asked me a series of routine questions, I was completely lucid and answered them from a profound depth of consciousness. I watched as my words seemed to bounce off his mind. I imagined him thinking, "Another patient on an anesthesia high." But I wasn't high, I was connected to the depths and fullness of my being. As I became aware of everyone scurrying around to check in on me, moving quickly up and down the corridor to attend to the needs of multiple patients, I felt sad for them. At heart they were empathic healers, but ones working in a mechanistic system that kept them in hurry mode and apt to operate on the surface. Despite these thoughts, I felt deep appreciation for their caring and tried to express that to them.

The sense of well-being from this anesthesia-induced and pranayama-assisted experience of pratyahara stayed with me for a few days. It made the reality of the yogic koshas (sheaths) undeniable, not as a model on paper, but in the living truth of my being. I can still summons this sense of being deeply centered in the Self, and surrounded by all the layers that comprise my body-mind, just by recalling the loveliness of that light and my time in the recovery room.

BE A DISCERNING STUDENT

Swami Kripalu saw pratyahara as the byproduct of a successful pranayama practice. But the ashram's teachings linking asana and pratyahara are also helpful. Attuning inward while doing postures leads to a state of inner focus that paves the way for the deeper experience of pratyahara that often occurs spontaneously while relaxing in corpse pose (shavasana) at the end of a yoga class. Often this experience is referred to by a different name—*yoga nidra* which literally means "yogic sleep"—but it is closely related to pratyahara. Swami Kripalu encouraged students to progress beyond this experience of deep relaxation in corpse pose by learning how to bring the same degree of bodily ease and inner absorption into their seated breathwork and meditation practice in a teaching he captioned: *There is no Entry into Meditation without Pratyahara.*

Pratyahara is the gateway to what the yogic sages call meditation. Once a seeker enters pratyahara, the remaining stages of dharana, dhyana and samadhi will unfold in due course. People tend to think that meditation only requires control of the mind. There is truth in this perspective, but if they fail to understand that introversion of the sense organs is also necessary for quieting the mind, they are making a mistake. The mind is not so simple and sane as to become easily absorbed in any single object of meditation. Until it is weaned away from the externalized sense organs by pranayama, the mind will remain constantly distracted. New stimulation will keep flowing in from outside, triggering chains of related thoughts.

Fighting inner and outer distractions simultaneously leaves little scope for victory. The yogis learned through hard experience that the mind cannot be made steady without the practice of pratyahara. This is why the Bhagavad Gita likens the mind to an impenetrable fort protected by the might of its encircling senses. Only after gaining control over these outposts can this fort be conquered, which is to say that only after pratyahara does the mind become fit for meditation.

APPLYING THIS CHAPTER IN PRACTICE

Each day before dinner, Danna and I do a simple practice that often elicits the experience of pratyahara, which we have come to call "conscious oblivion." We do a little yoga stretching to release the day's physical tensions, and then lie in corpse pose and begin a flowing breath. For several minutes we connect the inbreaths and outbreaths, shifting as smoothly as possible from one to the next, to create an uninterrupted flow of connected breathing. Before long the outside world falls away for a while, allowing us to deeply relax and return to our evening meal refreshed. Whenever Danna looks at me afterward and says, "I left," its apparent to me that she is emerging from the second stage of pratyahara.

Here is SK's guidance on how to bridge your practice of postures and yoga nidra with the more-conscious technique of sitting meditation, which he captioned *The Ritual of Pratyahara.*

In his book, Sage Goraksha instructs us: "Just as the evening sun slowly withdraws its light from the world, the meditating yogi should gradually withdraw the mind from the senses and turn it toward the soul." He then tells us how this can be accomplished: "In an orderly fashion, the five objects of sense perception (sight, sound, smell, touch, and taste) should be abandoned by the five sense organs (eyes, ears, nose, skin, and tongue). The condition that results is called pratyahara." This instruction should be carefully studied until it is well-understood.

When the sun rises and you open your eyes, all sorts of images and other sensations begin to enter your mind. During the day, an unceasing flow of sensory impressions occurs that can be likened to a constant tossing of pebbles into a still body of water that keeps its surface continually rippled. As a result, your mind is likely to grow disturbed. It is to return stillness to the mind that a yogi practices pratyahara.

Begin with the sense organ that seems easiest to you. Since sight and sound are the greatest disturbers of the mind, these are the senses attractive to beginners. In the effective practice of pratyahara, the eyes are usually shut. Refuge is taken in a secluded place, and any sounds coming from outside are ignored. After achieving pratyahara of the eyes and ears, the mind will automatically begin to withdraw its energy from the rest of the senses. Do not concern yourself with the problem of sequence. Just allow all the sense faculties to gradually grow quiet and introverted.

In conducting this ritual of pratyahara, you must remain aware that the mind is fickle and the sense organs are frivolous. The mind craves sensual stimulation, and the urge to return to the senses is very strong. A momentary slip is enough to distract and disturb the attention. Progress along this interior path can only be made by one who is patient and able to tolerate many disturbances.

He closed this teaching by posing and answering an important question that links the practice of pratyahara to the subsequent stages of yoga.

What is the difference between pratyahara and meditation? Pratyahara is a lower form of meditation. In pratyahara, quieting the sense organs is primary and steadying the mind is secondary. Knowing this distinction, all efforts are directed to making the sense organs introverted. In meditation, steadying the mind is primary and quieting the sense organs is secondary, so all efforts are directed to making the mind steady and introspective. The science of yoga teaches us that only after the state of pratyahara is reached can a yogi effectively practice dharana and eventually dhyana. If the techniques of these stages are attempted without first achieving pratyahara, they will not be able to carry us to the soul. This is why it is said that one must earn the right to practice dharana by achieving pratyahara.

While attending a Kripalu Center conference on the science of yoga, I heard a speaker anecdotally recount a research study involving a Zen roshi, a few Christian nuns, a yogi, and several members of a control group. Everyone was hooked up to instruments that measured their brain activity. While they were meditating, praying, or for the control group just sitting there, a starter's pistol was unexpectedly fired in the room. The brain activity of the control group immediately shot up and then remained high for quite a while as they recovered from the shock. The brain activity of the Zen roshi and Christian nuns also shot up, but then quickly returned to baseline, reflecting their ability to return to the present moment. The brain activity of the yogi never registered the shot, a fact that went unexplained by the speaker, but one I attributed to the phenomenon of pratyahara.

A yogic aspirant embarks on the inward journey to atman by quieting the mind. He knows that he can do this by becoming stable in any comfortable asana and closing the eyes. Aware that the mind will remain prone to distraction until the highly-perceptive sense organs are introverted, he understands that next he must perform pranayama until the senses grow introvert and the mind steadies enough to enter meditation. But the mere acceptance of these principles is not enough. An intent aspirant finds ways to regularly put them into practice.

CHAPTER 14

DHARANA

Yogic meditation is meant to be done methodically. An aspirant practices dharana in order to focus divergent streams of thought toward a single object of contemplation. In daily life, dharana bestows one's thoughts and actions with the power of undividedness. In yoga sadhana, it is dharana that concentrates the mind and renders it one-pointed and fit to practice the subsequent stage of dhyana, which alone is true meditation.

Dharana—focusing and fixating the mind on a single object of contemplation—is simple in both theory and application. A degree of self-discipline is required to undertake its practice, but there is not much ambiguity about what to do, or how to do it. Dharana is challenging only because it requires a direct confrontation with the restlessness of our own mind. While perhaps more prevalent in today's digital world, mental agitation is not a modern problem, as reflected in this centuries-old exchange between a yogic aspirant, Arjuna, and his guru, Krishna.

> Arjuna: This yoga you are teaching me requires an evenness of mind. The mind is unstable, Krishna, powerful, turbulent, inconstant, impetuous, self-willed, harassing, and always creating trouble. To control the mind seems as difficult to me as mastering the mighty winds.
>
> Krishna: Without a doubt, Arjuna, yoga is difficult to attain. For the mind is indeed restless and hard to restrain. Yet by steady practice the mind can be trained,

> if one knows the proper means, and if one works to apply them. (Bhagavad Gita 6:34)

Dharana is often translated as *concentration*, but technically-speaking that's not accurate. Dharana is derived from the Sanskrit root *dha*, which means *to hold*. Dharana is focusing your attention on a single point and holding it there, which over time strengthens your mind's capacity to concentrate. The goal of practice is not to stop the flow of thought, but to direct and steady it. In true dharana, all restless thoughts cease and even normal bodily awareness falls away, enabling all of your mental attention to stream in the direction of your chosen object of contemplation without any of its power being siphoned off in distraction.

It is easy to shift your attention to any one of the prescribed bodily points (adharas). Nor is it hard to direct your inner gaze to focus there. It is not even arduous to establish your attention firmly enough that the life energy begins to flow to that part of the body. But it is very difficult to firmly fix your awareness there until the mind becomes single-pointed and the vitality of that part blossoms. If you can learn to hold your attention unwavering, it will steadily replace the shallowness of your ignorance, which always leads to misery, with the depth of direct knowing, which always leads to greatness.

Before practicing dharana, an object of contemplation must be selected to serve as a target upon which to focus your attention. The best-known traditional word for this target is *alambana*, which means "supporting base or foundation."[1] An alambana can be a material object like a candle flame, the bodily process of breathing, a sacred set of words or mantra, a specific point or region of the body like the heart center, a geometrical diagram or *yantra*, or the visualized form of a deity. Once this target is chosen, the task is to focus your attention upon it and hold it steadily there. Don't imagine this will be easy. Expect the mind to resist your efforts and continue its habit of wandering. But if you persist, the

[1] Alambana is the term used in the Yoga Sutra for one's chosen object of meditation. Swami Kripalu preferred the word *adhara*, a Tantric term that means *a base for the practice of dharana*. Alambana is a broader term that continues to have relevance in the later limbs of dhyana and samadhi.

mind will gradually accustom itself to the practice. As the power of your dharana grows, all of your mental activity including your distractedness will begin to orbit around your alambana. Eventually the scattered mind can be focused like a magnifying glass, and pleasant periods of time will pass when its restlessness abates.

In the Yoga Sutra, Patanjali describes dharana: "When the pure mind is kept focused in the desired desa (region), it is called dharana." There are three traditional regions. The first consists of material objects. The second consists of subtle objects including the chakras and ideas or images held in the mind. The third is the divine region that includes celestial objects (sun, moon, etc.), various deities, and ultimately the living self (atman). The seeker may choose an object of contemplation from any one of these three regions on which to focus the mind. The mind easily becomes fixed on an object or idea if one has a great liking for it, so in dharana the predisposition of one's intellect and emotions play an important role.

A subsidiary form of mental constraint is practiced while doing asanas and pranayama, but when a yogi reaches the stage of dharana it is best to focus the mind on the bodily points (adharas), the energy centers (chakras), or the respective gods and goddesses said to indwell these chakras. At first the attention will not be able to remain steady for very long. But as the seeker advances in the practice of dharana, the mind will become capable of staying within the desired region for longer periods of time. This will cause prana to flow and become steady in the bodily part or chakra upon which you are concentrated, which in turn further steadies the mind.

Swami Kripalu taught several different methods for entering dharana. While he never linked them into a progression, they offer a set of increasingly-subtle techniques that can be practiced in succession to develop mastery in dharana.

DHARANA THROUGH PRAYER

SK's favorite way of entering dharana as a prelude to meditation was heartfelt prayer, which was the starting point he recommended for everyone. Non-theists can "pray" in this manner as demonstrated by the various invocations recited by Buddhist practitioners. Even purely secular approaches to meditation generally start with some affirmation or positive expression of intention to orient practice.

Great beings have revealed many ways of attaining dhyana (meditation), but the secret and most effective avenue is prayer. Prayer fixes the attention on a single task and results in a concentrated mind. Therefore, it is included in dharana. Genuine prayer is not possible until the senses have turned inward by the sentiment of devotion and their instinctive outward pull has subsided, therefore it includes pratyahara. It can be said that the realm of meditation begins where the boundary of prayer ends.

One who recites prayers from religious books does ordinary prayer. Praying in this way tends to be mechanical and often becomes boring. When rote prayers are recited with genuine affection, they become prayers of the medium order. This intermediate form of prayer is important. In the same way that a hot iron burns anyone who touches it, genuine prayer uplifts a person's character. It draws poison from the mind, revenge from the heart, and bitterness from the tongue.

The best prayer springs from a heart opened by the key of an inwardly focused mind. This prayer leaves one calm and composed because strength, peace, enthusiasm, and accurate knowledge from the intuition have been gained. With the spiritual appetite whetted, the moment has become ripe. It is this climax of prayer that brings one to the stage of meditation.

CONTEMPLATION OF THE BODILY POINTS

Next came the technique of focusing on the *bodily points* or *adharas*. In the contemporary world of yoga and Buddhism, this practice is often called a *body scan*.

In the Ramayana, the valiant Hanuman crosses the ocean in a single leap. Ordinary monkeys like us cannot do that. We need an incremental path to overcome the mind's impulsivity, which is why dharana should first be performed on gross objects. In the preliminary practice of tratak,[2] *the gaze is focused on the flame of a candle or lamp, a beautiful jewel, the statue of a deity, a picture of a saint or guru, or a potent mystical symbol. Material objects like this can provide the support we need to focus our attention and become acquainted with dharana. Systematic dharana practice can then begin by contemplating the eighteen vital points of the body. These are the big toes, ankles, calves, knees, thighs, anus, perineum, genitals, navel, heart, back, neck, throat, palate, nose, mid-point between the eyebrows, forehead and crown of head. This contemplation can be done either sitting or lying down and is performed like a meditation, where you start with the big toes and progress upwards to the crown of the head. At each vital point, you must steady the attention on that part of the body, and direct the prana (breath energy) to accumulate there, in order to achieve the necessary concentration of mind. The practice of ascending the staircase of the eighteen points can be trusted to strengthen dharana. And upon reaching the top, it will introduce you to dhyana (meditation).*

DHARANA ON THE ELEMENTS

The body scan leads seamlessly into the next technique, in which the definition of an *adhara point* is broadened to include a defined region of the body.

A more subtle form of dharana can be practiced on the five major elements. Yoga science teaches that the human body is made up of the five mahabhutas: earth, water, fire, air and ether. Each of them is described as governing a specific region of the body. The region from the big toes to the thighs is governed by the earth element. The region between the thighs and navel is governed by the water element. The region extending from the navel to the heart is governed

[2] Tratak is one of the six shat kriyas, see Appendix 4.

by the fire element. The region from the heart to the center of the eyebrows is governed by the air element, and the region above the eyebrows to the crown of the head is governed by the ether element. In this dharana (contemplation), the prana energy is focused on the lowest element and then progressively raised to the next element to gain control of the mind. Just as a forked stick is used to catch a powerful snake, the breath is made to flow steadily in each region of the body, and the fixated attention used to stabilize the prana energy there. Through the repeated practice of this dharana, one gradually attains command of the mind, which is conquered and rendered harmless by the ascending prana.[3]

DHARANA ON THE CHAKRAS

Swami Kripalu was confident that anyone established in concentrated inner awareness would eventually discover the chakras by sensing them as active points within their own energy field. In accord with this thinking, he generally refrained from instructing new students to focus on the chakras. Instead, he guided them to do pranayama along with the preliminary practices of dharana until they found the chakras for themselves by simply noticing what is already there. If and when this happens, practicing dharana on each of the chakras opens a doorway into an inner world. Swami Kripalu was careful to caution students that this stage of self-exploration was not without risks.

The mind of an advancing yogi established in dharana may become fixed on the various energy centers of the subtle body. Yoga science teaches that there are seven major chakras and three constricting granthis, and it is only through dharana and introspection that they can be known. Although the task of discovering the energy centers can be aided by studying their descriptions, it should be remembered that only encouragement is obtained from such study. Their

[3] In advanced forms of this contemplation, one inwardly or outwardly chants the seed mantra for each element while focusing on its respective bodily region, those mantras being: lam, vam, ram, yam, and ham. A version can be done utilizing postures targeted to activate each of the chakras – see page 5.

secrets can only be obtained through deep contemplation and systematic practice. As the mind begins to coalesce and steady, different obstacles may arise to divert a seeker from the path. The mind may be attacked by obsessive thoughts about some old, shameful, disturbing, or incomplete experience. Streams of illusory thoughts may arise in anticipation of some desirable experience to be had in the future. Fearful or beatific visions may arise. Some portraits of the Buddha show him meditating surrounded by a harem of maidens and monstrous figures to depict these difficulties. All such experiences should be regarded as the mind tempting us to step off the path of dharana so it may find relief in distraction.

THE RESULTS OF DHARANA

SK believed the practice of dharana would produce outcomes that enhanced one's life effectiveness and served as indicators of spiritual progress:

The effects of dharana are not imaginary—they are real. Dharana decreases the fluctuations of the mind, which fragments and dissipates its power. No sooner is the stage of dharana mastered than the yogi becomes decisive, skillful in his or her actions, and revered by other people. The power of dharana can be rightly utilized by a yogi but it must never be misused. A mind unified by dharana is alone the medium through which one can enter the most important internal spheres of yoga (dhyana and samadhi). It is also through dharana that sudden understanding can arise about the mystical secrets of life as enshrined in all the religions. It is at this stage that various siddhis (powers) can be gained. The true seeker is neither distracted by the profundity of their insights nor enslaved by siddhis. They use dharana to perfect their concentration, enter dhyana, and obtain direct spiritual knowledge in samadhi.

AN EXPERIENCE OF DHARANA

It's embarrassing to admit that I'd been meditating more than two decades before I was properly introduced to the power of dharana. It was 2003, and Danna and I were taking part in Kripalu Center's annual Yoga & Buddhism conference. The conference was directed by Stephen Cope, who in the ashram was known by his yoga name Kavi. Kavi told everyone on opening night that our days would begin before breakfast in the Main Chapel with an hour-long meditation led by Larry Rosenberg, a senior Buddhist teacher and the founder of the Cambridge Insight Meditation Center.

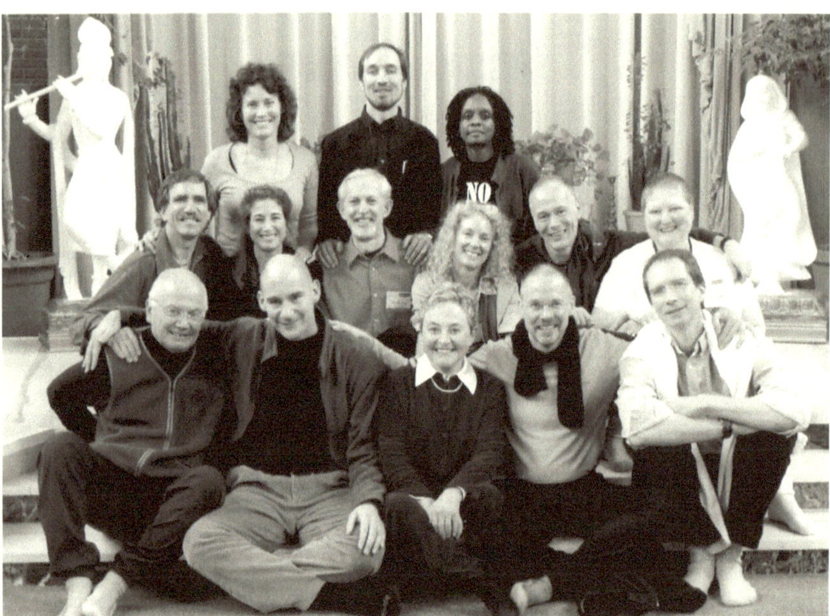

The Yoga & Buddhism faculty, with Larry Rosenberg sitting on the left-end of the front row, and Steven Cope the third person to his right. Steven was given the yoga name Kaviraj, which means "king of the poets," years before his potential as a writer emerged , and his life reflects all the attributes and achievements of a yogi cultivating what SK calls a partial kundalini awakening.

Larry came to the podium and explained that he would be training us in anapanasati, the primary form of meditation taught by the historical Buddha. Anapanasati remains the core practice of Theravadin and Zen Buddhism, and plays a prominent role in Tibetan Buddhism. It is also the basis of countless contemporary approaches to meditation in which it is translated to mean "mindfulness of breathing." Larry ended by saying that he would be teaching us the technique in its traditional form, where it is practiced as a means to cultivate the Seven Factors of Enlightenment that lead to equanimity, the release from dukkha (suffering), and the realization of nirvana.

I was taken by Larry's soft-spoken manner and internally made a commitment to participate fully in his training. The next morning arrived with Danna and me sitting on the floor of the Main Chapel shortly before 6:00 and ready to go. We'd gotten up early to do our posture and pranayama practice prior to the group meditation. Larry explained that for the next five mornings we would be focusing completely and exclusively on the breath. We would start by simply watching the breath. If an individual breath was long, we were told to mentally notice that the breath was long. If a breath was short, we were to mentally notice that the breath was short. This mindfulness of inhalation and exhalation was the foundation of the practice and had to be stringently developed.

Larry rang a small gong and the meditation began. Every few minutes, he would ask us, "Are you mindful of the breath? If your mind has wandered, bring it back by noticing if each breath is short or long." By the end of the session, I felt like jumping out of my skin. I'd not been able to go deep in meditation at all. Any time I started dipping beneath the surface of the thinking mind, Larry's voice pulled me back. I immediately told Danna, "The only way I can survive this is to get up really early so I can meditate on my own before doing yoga with you." Danna wasn't interested in getting up at 3:30, but she was fine with me doing so.

The next morning Larry started out by saying, "Over time, this meditation connects the mind and breath, making you sensitive to your entire body. Anchored by the breath, you will become aware of all your mental processes, and see first-hand how the body and mind are constantly changing." I relaxed, thinking that yesterday's session was introductory and today's practice would be quieter and deeper. But the way he led the meditation didn't shift an iota. I found the hour insufferable and walked out of the Main Chapel angry at Larry for "talking at us" the whole time. While eating our silent breakfast, Danna wrote me a note asking if she could borrow my ear plugs tomorrow.

The following morning, I resigned myself to doing the meditation on Larry's terms. He began by saying, "This morning the practice is going to shift a little. We are going to use the concentration we've built up to deepen our mindfulness." This sounded promising, but the first half of the meditation was a carbon copy of the previous days. But then Larry directed us to narrow our focus to the spot where the breath enters and leaves the nostrils. "Some of us might sense this at the tip of the nostrils," he said. "Others might feel the breath lightly striking an area of the upper lip." Either way, we were told to focus there and not let our awareness wander for even a second.

Thirty minutes later everyone was heading off to breakfast, but I sat there, unable to move. Fixating on that point, everything else in my mind had disappeared. I had not gone deep, as in entering another state of consciousness. But for a time, it seemed that my thought stream had come to a halt. I wasn't sure what exactly had happened, only that it had obviously affected me.

We repeated this practice the next day, and again I was able to narrow my focus and then bolt it down at this spot, which occurred to me as a tiny point of light. The steadiness of mind that resulted was something I had never experienced before. On the last day of the conference, Larry did loosen up his instructions. He began with a single sentence, "Gradually but with firm determination, become mindful of the breath." In the fifteen minutes that followed, he hardly said a word. In the quiet of the Main Chapel, I felt a soothing intimacy with my own breath. He then encouraged us to "sense the energy behind the breath," an invitation that ushered me into the kind of spacious state that up to then I'd associated with meditation.

During the conference, Larry and I were involved in some panel discussions, and there was good rapport between us. But only in this last meditation did I become grateful for the week of bootcamp mindfulness training he had given me. Walking to the front of the chapel, I was able to warmly thank him and start a dialogue that ended in us becoming friends.

BE A DISCERNING STUDENT

Back home from the conference, I felt thrown for a loop. For years I had used Swami Kripalu's basic meditation instructions—which included prayer, pranayama, and inner witnessing—to move through the stage of dharana and into a range of meditative states that characterize the next limb of yoga: dhyana. But now I'd been clearly shown there were profound states of concentrated attention unknown to me. Should I set aside my normal meditation protocol to delve deeper into dharana? Only when confronted by this dilemma did I come to understand a point that Swami Kripalu made repeatedly, and one essential to render the practice of yoga revelatory. *Sage Patanjali refers to the stages of dharana, dhyana, and samadhi by a single term—samyama—because they must be mastered together.*

Contemporary scholars support this view: "Samyama is the synergistic practice of dharana (fixation), dhyana (meditation), and samadhi (union). By locking the mind on a material or imagined object, fixation sharpens perceptual acuity and results in an effortless flow of concentrated awareness called meditation. Although these practices are given different names and sequentially related, they are integral parts of a single and continuous process of stilling the mind and achieving Self-realization."[4]

Over the next few months, it became clear to me that yogic meditation is meant to be practiced in layers. The process begins with asana—a stable seat that enhances bodily awareness. It continues with pranayama—steady and rhythmic breathing to quiet the senses and induce pratyahara. It culminates in the progression of dharana, dhyana, and samadhi, which I started to think of in simple terms as *focus, flow, and let go of all technique.* Once I understood the continuity of this process, it was easy to dedicate a little more time and energy to the layer of dharana, which I found deepened my dhyana.[5]

APPLYING THIS CHAPTER IN PRACTICE

Every year in early March, Kavi remedied his Massachusetts winter doldrums by spending a month at the vacation home of a family friend in

[4] Excerpted from *The Roots of Yoga*: pages 283-286.

[5] Anyone practicing dharana should understand that narrowing and focusing the beam of attention activates the sympathetic nervous system. This produces an uptick in energy that increases one's ability to concentrate upon a single point. But if done too stringently, or for prolonged periods of time, as often done in a retreat setting, this can overstimulate the nervous system and lead to adverse effects – see the work of Willoughby Britton, PhD, and cheetahhouse.org. In a mature meditation practice, the initial energy boost provided by dharana is used to move into the open-monitoring of dhyana, which provides a parallel and balancing stimulation of the parasympathetic nervous system.

Key West, Florida. Not long after the conference, Kavi invited Danna and me to visit him for a week, staying in a tiny apartment behind the house whose bathroom was made complete by an outside shower. Each morning, we did our solo practices. During the day, Kavi wrote while we explored the town on bicycles. Freeloading off his rent, we were happy shopping for dinner. There was a hot yoga studio nearby with a flamboyant instructor and late afternoon class that Danna really enjoyed. Afterward, we'd get cleaned up and start cooking. Kavi joined us in the kitchen around 6:30, and the three of us would meditate for an hour in the living room, after which we would eat and share the evening.

Kavi was researching a book on the Yoga Sutra that would later be published as *The Wisdom of Yoga*. On Saturday evening, all three of us were feeling the impending breakup of the happy little molecule we'd formed. This led Kavi to remark, "I've had all sorts of friends visit, but hardly any willing to meditate the way we have. I don't get it – nothing is as compelling to me as the process of sitting down, settling in, and gathering awareness until it coalesces and begins to stream toward a single point. And doing it together, even when each of us is doing our own thing, you can feel our minds entraining. Why am I so alone in this?"

I immediately recognized this utterance as highly influenced by all the time he was spending with the Yoga Sutra. I still recall the fascinating discussion that followed. By the end of the evening, the three of us had arrived at our best explanation. A lot of people meditate, but few persevere through the stage of dharana, where the scattershot mind begins to shine with an inner light. Standing around the kitchen as the dishes got done, Kavi was glowing and gave voice to his inspiration. "A big part of why people don't reach the stage of dharana has nothing to do with their commitment or even the regularity of their practice. It's that they don't adequately understand the stages of meditation. That's what I want to explain in this book, in a way that everyone can understand." As they say, the rest is history.

Dharana, dhyana, and samadhi. These three are inseparable, constituting an integral whole. Sage Patanjali calls this trio "samyama" and tells us exactly how to practice them. Having withdrawn the mind from the sense organs, a seeker must focus their attention on an object of contemplation and concentrate upon it such that nothing else exists in their consciousness. Through this practice alone, the seeker's mind will enter dhyana and pass through various meditative states before attaining the super-consciousness of samadhi. Sage Patanjali assures us, "By mastering samyama, the highest wisdom is attained." This explains why it can be said that dharana is the seed; dhyana is the tree, and samadhi is the fruit.

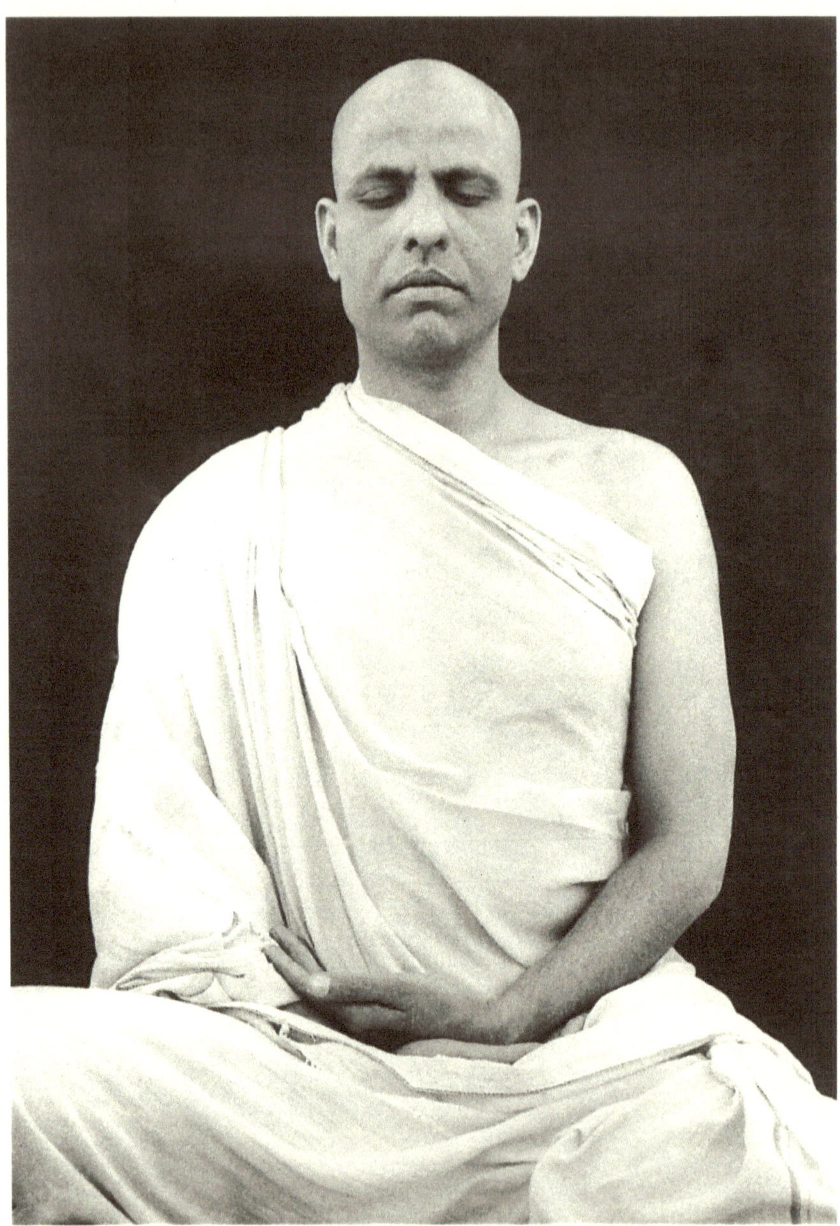

SK practicing awareness-focusing meditation in his early years as a swami, before his kundalini awakened fully and his and practice of energy-raising meditation began.

CHAPTER 15

DHYANA

It is not possible to gain knowledge of your superior nature without the regular practice of meditation, which yoga calls dhyana.

The ashram's dawn-to-dark schedule of mandatory activities did not include much time for sitting meditation. Lots of things were done meditatively. Work periods began with a centering. Community gatherings were preceded by chanting and dancing. Morning and afternoon yoga sessions were aimed at doing postures as meditation-in-motion and ended with a few unstructured minutes to lie or sit. As helpful as all these activities were in the effort to stay present and attuned, none of them provided the regular opportunity to rest in stillness that is required for the mind to not only momentarily settle but steadily be refined. Studying his teachings, it's hard for me not to think that Swami Kripalu would have done things differently.

Meditation is integral to yoga. Because people are different, various approaches to meditation have evolved to suit their needs. Seekers should experiment with a variety of techniques until they find one to their liking. But if there is no meditation in the practice, it cannot be called yoga.

By the time Danna and I moved into the ashram in the late 1980s, the need for meditation was growing acute. One by one, residents began to sneak off to nearby retreat centers, using their vacation time to learn Vipassana meditation. Looking back, it's laughable that these Buddhist intensives were officially labelled "off limits" out of fear they might encourage residents to stray from their yogic path, especially when

Swami Kripalu's discourses are peppered with praise for what he called *Buddha dharma*. More to the point, the ashram's failure to incorporate sitting meditation into its yoga curriculum was keeping residents from exploring the breadth and depth of SK's teachings on dhyana, which can be applied to any form of meditation. This chapter aims to recover a bit of that loss.

Sage Patanjali tells us that all yogic seekers must withdraw their minds from the sense organs and fix their attention on an object of contemplation. After steadfastly concentrating upon it, they must patiently purify their mind by passing through the meditative states of dhyana on the way to the super-consciousness of samadhi. While this is universally true, people are of differing natures and inclinations. As a result, different approaches to attaining dhyana have evolved and seekers are free to choose the meditation technique that best meets their needs. While no single method of dhyana is for everyone, all seekers must adopt an approach that appeals to them and practice it methodically.

WHAT IS DHYANA?

Strictly speaking, dhyana is not a stage of yoga that can be practiced independently. Dhyana is a quality of mind that occurs when the prior stage of dharana becomes effortless. As taught in the Yoga Sutra, dharana is fixing the mind on one area, object, or idea. Dhyana results when the flow of concentrated attention toward that area, object, or idea becomes single and continuous. In other words, dhyana happens naturally as your practice of dharana matures. Traditional commentaries on this verse liken the current of awareness passing through the mind in dhyana to an unbroken stream of viscous oil being smoothly poured from one vessel to another. Thought continues to flow, but it is purposefully targeted and no longer experienced as dissipating or distracting.

It is true that flowing through the mind of a meditating yogi is a constant stream of thoughts, but it is equally true that this yogi is in a state of dhyana. Seekers who believe the mind should become thoughtless in meditation become disheartened when that does not happen. Sometimes a horse is allowed to graze in an open field while tethered by a long rope. The state of a seekers mind during dharana and dhyana is similar to the condition of this horse. Supportive thoughts close to your object of contemplation are cultivated, while thoughts farther afield are curbed. For one who knows this, accessing dhyana becomes easy and meditation begins to steadily purify the mind-stream of undesired and distracting thoughts. It is through this thought-winnowing that the seeker's mind is continually refined. As the state of one-pointed concentration (ekagrata) is approached, the impact of dhyana upon the mind becomes greater and greater.

Ordinarily, a thought-wave arises in the mind only to be erratically followed by a successive thought-wave moving in a different direction. In the practice of dhyana, the current of thought is made to flow continuously in one direction and with a singular intent. As the mind is suffused in a flow of synchronous thought, it gives rise to an inner experience of stillness and tranquility. This explains why the analogy of the steadily-poured oil is apt. The oil stream appears to be motionless, even though the oil comprising it is in constant motion. A modern metaphor is the laser beam, in which light rays are brought into phase to produce a beam of coherent light with waves of exactly the same wavelength. Yoga calls this state of mental coherence ekagrata (one-pointedness) and testifies to the laser-like power it brings to the mind.[1]

If you understand the stage of dhyana clearly, the basic tools of meditation that you are already practicing have the capacity to turn on the power of the mind. At your level of practice, you may not be aware that the refinement of the mind is the evolution of the person. As your mind-power develops, you cease to be dominated by the egocentric life of the senses. Your search for truth begins in earnest. In response, your intellect, your intuition, your ability to reason and analyze will go on increasing. Preparing to meditate,

[1] This phenomena of the seemingly-still but constantly moving oil stream fascinated early yogis and is called a tailadharavat. References to it appear in the Upanishads and the Vedantic teachings of Shankara.

you will be like the owner of a radio who turns the knob and sees the power light come on. Then you can adjust your mental radio dial to tune out all the static and disturbances and receive only the desired frequency. Do not think that this can be done in a single meditation session or you will be disappointed. You have to persist in your practice. But as you learn to use these tools effectively, and demonstrate the patience needed to bear the difficulties that inevitably arise to block progress, you will come to know the true power of the mind and increasingly receive the light of spiritual Self-knowledge.

Progressing from dharana into dhyana, you are likely to encounter a range of meditative states accompanied by shifts in bodily awareness, vivid emotions of all kinds, visual images, intuitive insights, and occasional moments of bliss or rapture. The practice is to simply be with each experience – whether pleasant, unpleasant, or neutral – allowing it to arise and pass through your awareness like clouds in the sky. If you become lost in story or distraction, simply come back to your object of contemplation to regain focus. Then gradually allow your awareness to once again broaden and flow. You will likely repeat this process of moving from dharana into dhyana multiple times in a single sitting. Ideally, meditation ends with a period in which you drop all technique and simply be. As much as possible, surrender any attempt to focus the mind or in any way manipulate your experience. Learn to rest in effortless being.

BENEFITS OF PRACTICE

Swami Kripalu saw meditation as intrinsically valuable. Very few therapies, life-enhancing products, or prescription drugs can legitimately claim to deliver an almost-immediate move toward greater self-awareness and peace of mind. Yet meditation does this, and in addition has a number of side benefits that SK felt were worth noting. Perhaps the most important of these is meditation's ability to increase creativity and improve the executive function of the mind.

Concentration is the secret to skillful action. The mind of an author, painter, musician, dancer, or orator is always one-pointed when creating their masterpiece. All the discoveries and inventions of science are likewise the result of profound and prolonged contemplation. Great leaders also have to pass through these stages of concentration in order to stand resolute before the people and courageously announce their decisions. Any expert, when asked how they achieved their goal, will answer, "through concentration." Together, such individuals have made a deep impression on society. Because concentration has been achieved by so many different individuals in so many areas of life, it indicates an ability that can be cultivated by anyone. After understanding the value of concentration, and comparing the various methods of steadying the mind, one will conclude that the eight-limbs of yoga and in particular the stages of dharana and dhyana are straightforward and scientific.

If we understand how meditation is intended to work, it also has the power to lift our mood and ratchet up the emotional set-point from which we habitually operate. With the rates of anxiety and depression spiking the world over, this is another of meditation's profound side benefits.

It appears that a meditator's mind becomes filled with joy. But in truth joy is the mind's very nature. Only when drawn into the strong currents of attraction and aversion does the mind become conflicted and miserable. A meditator remains neutral and observes the activities of the mind as a disinterested witness. As a result, the nervous system grows calm, and the meditator's mind lays down its burdens. It is in this quietude that the mind's innate joy becomes apparent. That is how the mind becomes elevated through the practice of dhyana.

Every regular meditator discovers that the benefits of meditation spill over into the rest of their life. SK considered daily life the true test of meditation mastery.

After years of practicing meditation, the process of dhyana becomes so natural that a yogi is able to remain tranquil under any condition. A task arises and the yogi concentrates the mind upon it. Appropriate thoughts are generated and prana enables the body to effectively carry out whatever actions are called for. While it's noteworthy when an aspirant's mind becomes peaceful in meditation, that aspirant can only be said to be a yogi when their mind remains peaceful outside the meditation room. After learning to ride a bicycle, one becomes able to cycle smoothly down a crowded street, even while conversing with a cycling companion. It is the same with a yogi and dhyana.

Swami Kripalu was a spiritual teacher and not an executive coach, psychologist, or counselor. In the final analysis, he valued the process of meditation taught by yoga as a time-tested means of awakening.

Everyone strives for worldly accomplishment but only a few genuinely seek spiritual advancement. Dhyana is the best means for purifying the thought-stream and preparing the mind for Self-realization by making it peaceful. Through its practice one begins to see that our being has its source in atman, which can be thought of as the principle of aliveness through which the body and mind are manifested. It is only through this insight into atman that our higher consciousness and superior nature can be awakened. At first this awakening only exists during periods of introversion and contemplation. Eventually it is based on the realization of the essence and not merely upon its contemplation.[2] *A ray of sunlight appears to be separate from the sun. But in truth the ray is not separate, as its origin is in the sun. Similarly, an individual soul appears to be separate from God or Brahman. But these two are not truly separate, as the soul remains connected to its divine source, and their essence is one and the same. Those seeking enlightenment should not undervalue the mental peace that is its essential prerequisite. Obtain it through dhyana, then use it to gain insight into atman.*

---

[2] The phrase "realization of the essence" is a shorthand reference SK used to refer to the discovery that your essence as an individual (atman) is not qualitatively different from the essence of ultimate reality (Brahman). He also used the term "having seen the equivalence" for this important insight – see page 219.

MEDITATION NIGHT

I took part in dozens of ashram yoga trainings and workshops. But truth be told, I learned more about dhyana from a weekly gathering of friends we called Meditation Night. It was hosted by one of our closest friends, Jonathan Foust, who was known in ashram circles by his Sanskrit name Sudhir. Sudhir was introduced to TM in prep school and has been meditating ever since. He moved into the ashram in 1981, hoping to immerse himself in his practice, and was surprised to find hardly anyone else interested in sitting still.

Sudhir and I met in the early 1980s, when Danna and I were bottom-tier but regular donors. He was our contact in the fundraising department. Sudhir and I got to know each other in the thick of the guru scandal in 1994, when he was in charge of public relations, and I was responsible for providing him accurate and up-to-date legal information. We became fast friends after I returned as Kripalu Center's president and hoodwinked him into serving as the vice president of curriculum.

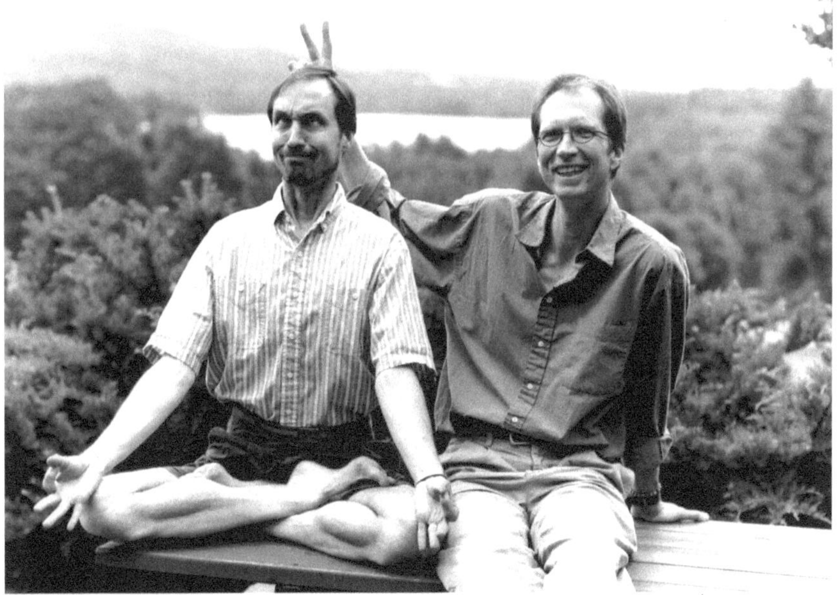

Sudhir and the author goofing off on the front steps of Kripalu Center during the years they were upper-level administrators.

Every Wednesday, a group of us gathered at 6:30 in Sudhir's living room to meditate for an hour. Each week we enacted the same ritual.

Sudhir got home early enough to put a half dozen monster yams in the oven. Danna would make a big vegetable casserole, and I would bake a pan of corn bread. For protein one of us always brought a tub of almond butter. With these dietary bases covered, the other attendees could fill in around the edges to make for a healthy potluck meal. We kept any upfront socializing to a minimum to get directly to meditation. After designating a timekeeper, we would sit for an hour. Then we'd fill plates and while eating go around the circle, with each person having an opportunity to share what was up in their life and practice. When the circle closed, we cleaned up and hightailed it home to get to bed early.

On the very first meditation night, something happened that bonded Sudhir, Danna, and me in this shared endeavor. Danna was the first to share and told a story from our early days as true believers. Like all the donors, we had received a guru-poster in the mail sporting an inspiring quote, which Danna recounted from memory: "Each day I affirm that there is nothing in this world that can stop me from transforming my life, opening my heart, loving myself, and sharing my love with everyone I encounter." After hanging the poster in our yoga room, we closed our morning meditation by gazing at the guru's smiling face and speaking this affirmation of his aloud for well-over a year. Danna ended her sharing by asking if she could ever recover that kind of faith with everything that had happened since. Listening intently, Sudhir chimed in. "Yeah, I remember that poster. But it wasn't really a guru quote – I wrote it." After a moment of stunned silence, the three of us laughed so hard that our tears for innocence lost mingled with the mirth of the moment. The full gestalt of the experience was quite healing.

In the next few sessions, a practical problem was solved in a way that taught all of us the difference between dharana and dhyana. Sudhir had a Standard Poodle named Hakuna who acted more human than canine. As everyone sat down to meditate, Hakuna would start going from person to person, nuzzling them to say hello and elicit a little attention. That led Sudhir to get a large bone with a little gristle left on it. Right before we started, he would give the bone to Hakuna in the adjoining room to occupy his attention.

For a few weeks, the first fifteen minutes of meditation was close to intolerable, as all of us struggled to concentrate our minds on anything but the sound of Hakuna's chewing. But around the 20-minute mark, we would emerge from the stages of pratyahara and dharana to enter dhyana. The sound seemed to fade into the background, and it ceased to be disturbing. As the weeks went by, we began to hardly notice the initial period of chewing, accepting it as Hakuna focusing on his "object of contemplation." The group sharing that followed the sitting was consistently rich and meaningful, so much so that none of us liked to miss a night.

Once we had a flow established, Sudhir started inviting any visiting teachers whom he felt were sympatico with our group. Some amazing discussions were sparked by the interface of meditation night regulars and outside luminaries. Becoming a skillful meditator requires expert instruction, especially to get started. And there is no way around the individual time on the cushion needed to learn how to work with your own mind. But a group of friends willing to support each other in sustaining a regular practice can be a real asset.

BE A DISCERNING STUDENT

Swami Kripalu taught that a yogi practicing dhyana will pass through a broad spectrum of mind-states, with each of them contributing in some way to their psychological growth and spiritual unfolding. This parallels the teaching of the Buddha, who taught in the Pali language, where the Sanskrit word dhyana becomes *jhana*. Buddha cataloged eighty-nine different states of consciousness, which were grouped into nine levels, each of which was called a jhana.[3]

First Jhana: Pleasant Sensations
Second Jhana: Joy
Third Jhana: Contentment
Fourth Jhana: Utter Peacefulness
Fifth Jhana: Infinity of Space
Jhana: Infinity of Consciousness
Seventh Jhana: No-thingness

[3] The first four jhanas are states resulting from focused concentration that roughly correspond to the yogic stage of dharana. The remaining five jhanas are called "formless absorptions" that seem to correspond to the yogic stages of dhyana and samadhi. Technical differences aside, it seems clear these maps are describing the same territory.

Eighth Jhana: Neither perception nor non-perception
Ninth Jhana: Cessation of all mental activity

SK used a comparable but lesser-known yogic model to depict this spectrum called the *samapattis*, which he defined as *the meditative states that lead to the correct (sama) acquisition of truth (apatti).*

There are four samapattis through which a seeker has to pass before reaching samadhi. Each is designated by a name that reflects the quality of mind prevalent in that level: deliberative, reflective, joyful, and Self-realized. The supporting object of meditation in the first three levels shifts from gross to subtle to very subtle. In the fourth level, the seeker meditates on the sense of self, leaving aside all other means of supporting the mind to know Self-realization, which is accompanied by a mind state mature enough to be identified as samadhi.

To counter the rosy labels attached to these levels in both the Buddhist and yogic models, Swami Kripalu cautioned against presuming that your progress through the samapattis and jhanas should be easy and uneventful. While the overall journey is meant to carry you in a good direction, it is wise to expect bumps in the road.

It should not be assumed from the names of the samapattis that a seeker's mental state won't continue to go up and down. At times you will feel inner happiness and joy. But you will also confront boredom, distractedness, encounter painful or frightening experiences, and endure times when total darkness seems to fall across your path. Even when the mind is perturbed or stupefied at how to overcome the hurdles needed to advance, it must be remembered that continuous self-awareness is what leads to an abiding samadhi.

It's noteworthy that psychology describes a similar spectrum of mind states under the umbrella term *metacognition*, which literally means "above cognition." Metacognitive development is a process that commences with the ability we all have to step outside the thought stream and observe its content. As that capacity expands, a person becomes increasingly aware of their mental patterns and able to monitor, evaluate, and to some extent control their thinking. This is known to improve learning, problem solving, and decision-making. It is also believed to enhance mental health.

Research has shown that experienced meditators activate the same areas of the brain that psychology associates with metacognitive awareness. Psychologists believe that meditators develop this awareness by tracking the movement of attention, simply noticing rather than mindlessly following where their thoughts and feelings would have them go. This lessens the salience generally attributed to what is happening in the foreground of the mind, and highlights the presence of its background awareness.

These psychologists go further to acknowledge two qualitatively different levels of experience. The first is our awareness of whatever object we are perceiving, which our ordinary mind state provides. The second is the metacognitive knowing that we are aware of that object in the present moment, which requires us to recognize our deeper identity as awareness itself. The parallels between these ideas and the teachings on samadhi provided by both Yoga and Buddhism are unmistakable. Both of these Eastern approaches teach that it's possible to see into the machinery of the mind to a depth that illumines a host of areas considered by psychology to be unconscious. The extent to which that is scientifically true remains unknown, but the meditation research already conducted makes it clear that developing metacognitive awareness enables us to see a significantly larger swath of our subconscious and often repetitive mental content. This is really nothing new. Western writings evidencing an understanding of metacognition date back to the ancient Greeks.

Cultivating a mix of metacognitive "wisdom" and empathic "compassion" was an essential element of traditional yoga and Buddhism. Contemporary Buddhism places a greater emphasis on the technique of *lovingkindness meditation* or *metta*, which provides psychologists with a simple compassion-building protocol to study. Research shows that awareness-focusing meditation and metta are qualitatively different techniques in terms of how they affect the brain. This suggests there is benefit to practicing not just one but both. Swami Kripalu adds the idea that there may be a link connecting them.

Once I admitted to my Gurudev, "Whenever I pray to God, I begin to cry." In response, he gave me a great teaching. "Crying is the outward expression of the pain in your heart," he said. "While it's true you are crying, you are crying for your own pain." This invited me to see that feeling my own pain was only a first step. The next step is to become like a caring mother or father, whose heart is touched by the cry of their child. Everyone's suffering should be heard by us as a heart-rending cry for attention. The final step is to cry out to the Lord with a pure heart moved by everyone's suffering and also feeling the pain of our own separation from the Divine. Nothing compares to the power of this wordless prayer. All the principles of yoga are included in it. One who arouses these feelings of compassion and devotion enough to know this crying knows yoga sadhana. Crying out for our own pain, we can fill our hands with tears and little will come of it. But if even a single drop is for the welfare of others, or stems from a pure yearning for the One, it will begin a process that destroys our egocentric intoxication and actualizes a hidden potential for love that will take over the mind and intellect, causing them both to fully develop.

APPLYING THIS CHAPTER IN PRACTICE

Practicing dhyana requires more than sitting down to meditate. Dhyana marks the culmination of yoga's earlier stages in which you learn to stabilize the position of the body, engage then steady the breath, introvert the senses, and focus the mind. A good meditation protocol enables you to touch all these bases and trigger a natural movement into dhyana. One of the traditional practices used to induce the experience of dhyana gives you a feel for the state itself. Sitting on a flat rock overlooking a wide river, an experienced yogi closes his eyes to concentrate the mind. After settling into meditation, he opens his eyes and simply watches the river flow by.

In 2003, Danna and I had the opportunity to lead daily yoga classes in support of a Vipassana Retreat at Spirit Rock Meditation Center. During the first two weeks, all the retreat participants were taught to enter dhyana by focusing on their breath and then performing a thorough body scan. In the evenings, one of the senior teachers would deliver a Dharma Talk. In the final talk of that two-week period, the marquis teacher boiled all the prior meditation instruction down to a simple maxim: *not too loose; not too tight.* While arguably a bit simplistic, I have found this trustworthy counsel. If my attention is loose enough to allow the mind to wander or become spacey, I will never overcome distraction and enter dharana. If my attention is overly tight and constricting, I will never be able to relax into dhyana.

For years, I practiced meditation trusting its ability to lead me down the path of yoga. And without a doubt, I was reaping the benefits of what Swami Kripalu called *a continual refinement of mind.* Sitting each morning, I watched all of my most difficult work-related and personal problems get resolved by insights that emerged from the process of going in and out of dhyana. Amazed by this experience, I came to think of open questions and unresolved issues like this as tensions in my mind. As the tension released, creative solutions reliably arose, provided my meditation was motivated by a sincere desire to connect spiritually and not to solve my problems. But eventually I began to suspect that all these meditative states were ultimately a tease. As the understanding slowly dawned that the mind is simply not equipped to know reality directly, it became increasingly clear that I needed something qualitatively different and yet unknown to continue moving forward.

The realm of nature is vast. In order to cross it and merge into atman, the domain of meditation must start with the material body and extend into the subtle layers of mind. In the late stages of dhyana, the respiratory system operates independently of mind. The inhalations and exhalations become so naturally slow and rhythmic that no movement of breath is registered in awareness. Inwardly the attention remains steady, but the mind becomes unable to concentrate on even the subtlest object of meditation. As a result, the mental field of the yogi becomes blank and void of any inclinations. It is at this point that samadhi is near.

CHAPTER 16

A GLIMPSE OF SAMADHI

In India, the study of one's own self is considered the direct route to realization. Traversing it, the question "Who am I?" is meditatively pondered. While the value of this practice may be hard to fathom, the yogis discovered that all the spiritual knowledge in the world can be obtained through it.

My friend Sudhir is an unusually creative guy and a great listener to boot. Back when I was Kripalu Center's president, the two of us were in constant contact as he helped me think through all the thorny issues facing the organization. But once a week the tables were turned in an hour-and-a-half meeting where I was his sounding board on curriculum matters. Sliding a single-page flyer across my desk, Sudhir gave me a run down on a retreat called The Enlightenment Intensive. "It's an experiential form of Advaita Vedanta that's been around since the sixties. Everything is based on a carefully-structured dyad technique in which partners go back and forth contemplating the question Who am I? It's a novel approach to self-inquiry that is highly relational, which dovetails nicely with how we do things. Participants report powerful, even life-changing experiences. If we decide to offer it here, it would be a three-night program scheduled over a holiday weekend."

"Okay, I responded, "It sounds interesting, but what about the name. Three days to enlightenment is serious hyperbole. What about the integrity of our marketing?" Sudhir had obviously anticipated this objection and was quick to respond. "The whole idea is this single technique, done repeatedly, has the power to break you free of all the mind's conditioning. From what I can tell the program has a good track record. As for the name, it's been called that for decades. I don't think we'd want to change it now." Satisfied and content to end the conversation, I continued. "Sudhir, I trust your judgment. It sounds like you've looked into this and concluded it's a good addition to our curriculum. You're in charge of your area and don't need my permission to schedule a new program. But if you're asking because this retreat is a little edgy, self-inquiry is part of yoga. That's our mission and you have my support."

"It's not that simple," Sudhir protested. "It's a serious intensive. The schedule goes from six in the morning to ten at night. For three days, the participants do this contemplation technique all day long, with short breaks for walks and portioned meals. Before we can promote this, I need to know it's safe for our guests, including first-timers. The only way for me to be certain is to take the intensive myself. To do that, I need a few days off and a little money for a road trip to Bar Harbor, Maine."

Now the issue was on the table. "Man, you work like a maniac. A few days off campus to check out a promising program is no problem." While saying this, I remembered that Accounting had stripped all the R&D money out of the Programs department to make the budget work. Opening a three-ring binder, I made sure my Administration department had the funds. "If $750 will cover your expenses, sign yourself up." Sudhir was not done yet. "Thanks for the green light, but I'm not finished my due diligence. I'll keep you posted."

Turning our attention to the next agenda item, I had no inkling that this conversation heralded a turning point in my life—and Danna's even more so.

The ancient yogis believed there is knowledge hidden in the innermost aspect of a person, which we call the soul and they called atman. It was in order to unlock the secrets of atman that they developed the techniques of svadhyaya, which means "the study of the self." Compiling the Yoga Sutra, sage Patanjali included self-study in his formulation of kriya yoga. In this approach, intensive self-investigation is done after preliminary disciplines to purify the body and mind (tapas) and before the start of surrender meditation (Ishvara pranidhana). From this point of view, svadhyaya is one of yoga's three major tools for growth.

OUR FIRST INTENSIVE

As his potential road trip drew near, Sudhir became convinced of the program's value. Before firming up his reservation, he made a pitch for me and Danna to go with him. "I'm driving up anyway. If you two pay your tuition, it will be a cheap vacation." That evening, I described the intensive to Danna certain she would be dead set against taking part. To my great surprise, she immediately opted in and told me, "I'm no candidate for enlightenment, but I'm willing to accompany you and Sudhir on the expedition." At the time, the intensive presented a rare opportunity to get me away from my desk. Having so little time together, she must have known that I would have never gone without her.

Arriving in Bar Harbor, it quickly became apparent the Enlightenment Intensive we were taking was an intimate affair. Sixteen participants, a single teacher, and two helpers occupied what was once a sprawling farmhouse. The retreat activities took place on the second floor of a small adjacent outbuilding. One of the assistants was Missy Hatch, a talented chef whom I happened to know well from the 1980s when the two of us had taken Kripalu Yoga Teacher Training together. Her exquisite meals were served in modest, plated portions to keep everyone alert and attentive.

Otherwise, the retreat was much as Sudhir had described save one notable exception. The question "Who am I?" was turned into a directive that made it a potent instruction: "Tell me who you are." Sitting in pairs or "dyads," we went back and forth on this inquiry in five-minute increments after which a gong would sound. For five minutes, one person would be the "contemplating partner" and the other would be the "listening partner." When the gong sounded, the roles would switch. Doing this four times resulted in a forty-minute "Enlightenment Exercise" after which a louder and longer gong would ring to signal its end.

Once I got the hang of the technique, it didn't take long to feel the power of this partner-assisted method of self-inquiry. It was doubly potent to witness the work of all the other participants as they cycled through their biographical data and family of origin stories, vividly recounting past events pivotal to their self-concept. By the end of the second day, we'd dug down to shed light on our most neurotic patterns, and risen up to give voice to our grandest notions, and it was growing increasingly clear that in truth we were none of this thought-based mind content. Repeatedly receiving the instruction from my partner, "Tell me who you are," I found myself with less and less to say. Taking the place of all my discarded mental clutter was a growing sense of clarity and inner spaciousness.

Not knowing what else to do, I fell back on my experience as a meditator. Drawing close to the mysterious source of my being, I held my attention there, basking in its proximity but unable to break through the "barrier of pure consciousness" to what the intensive calls "a direct experience of self, not mediated by the mind." I felt like a stack of dry wood, the entirety of my being calling out for an inner spark or lightning strike. And on day three the lightning strike came, but it hit Danna instead. For the rest of the day, she was a live wire, more animated and joyous than I had ever seen her.

When the gong clanged to end the final dyad, it was clear that I'd struck out swinging at enlightenment. But in the process, I had learned something incredibly important. My meditation practice had carried me through a multitude of increasingly subtle mind states. Exactly as Swami Kripalu promised, it had purified my thought stream and refined my cognitive capacities. But the intensive had shown me that meditation—as I was practicing it then—was ultimately dead-ended. There is no incremental way to know the Infinite. A different tool was needed to break out of the dualistic mind and experience the unified Self directly.

Sudhir and I had both thrown ourselves into the retreat. Exhausted, we took turns driving back to the Berkshires while needling Danna, who couldn't stop saying all sorts of profundities in lyrical verse. Unlike us, she was wide-awake, but in no condition to pilot Sudhir's minivan down I-95. When things got quiet, I thought deeply about the intensive. While simple in theory, there was genius reflected in its crisp technique and supportive structure. Inwardly, I vowed to learn everything there was to know about it.

I returned to a backlog of emails and meeting requests longer than both my arms. But that didn't stop me from looking into the history of the intensive while the experience was still fresh. What I found with a simple computer search made my jaw drop. Staring wide-eyed at my monitor, I phoned Danna. When she picked up, I stammered out what was on the screen. The intensive was created in 1968 by Charles Berner, a name that obviously hadn't rang a bell for Sudhir. But I knew that Charles Berner was also known as Yogeshwar Muni, the chief American disciple of Swami Kripalu. It was Berner's California ashram that had offered and popularized the Enlightenment Intensive. This retreat, which had affected both Danna and me so strongly, was yogically-speaking a branch off our family tree.

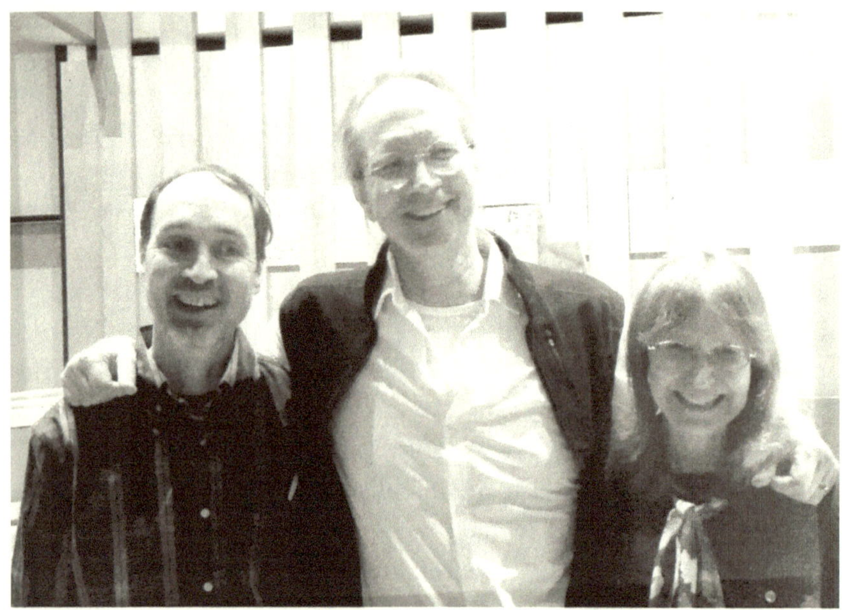

The friendship born in Meditation Night and forged in the Enlightenment Intensive led Sudhir, Danna, and the author to offer a yoga, breathwork, and meditation program called the Energy Intensive that ran for 20 years at Kripalu Center.

MORE INTENSIVES

Sudhir's effort to integrate the Enlightenment Intensive into Kripalu Center's curriculum enabled Danna to take a half dozen of them over the next six months. I was able to do four, including one offered gratis to the staff. Right off the bat in our first intensive, Danna and I took to the inquiry process like ducks to water. In these subsequent ones, each of us found that the power of the technique did not wane with repetition. To the contrary, its impact increased as we began working with a different directive, "Tell me what you are," which is a more-targeted pointer to one's true nature.

During this time, I read *The Enlightenment Intensive: Dyad Communication as a Tool for Self-Realization.* It was authored by Lawrence Noyes, a close student of Berner carrying on this work after their ashram's demise, which made me think the two of us might have lots in common. When I learned that Lawrence was offering a ten-day training in how to lead intensives that summer, I signed up. Within a few months, I was on my way to meet him in Toronto. On the first day of the training, I was given a hefty two-volume manual written in a pragmatic voice that was truly instructive. It detailed all the ins and outs of the dyad technique, and a refined mental model of what enlightenment is and isn't. Reading it twice cover to cover, I came to understand the barrier I was confronting in my meditation practice.

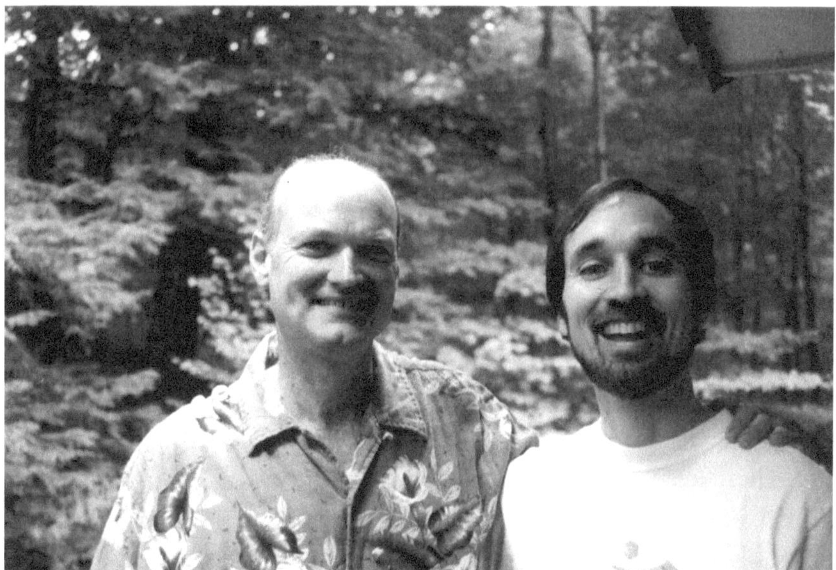

Lawrence Noyes and author in Toronto during the ten-day Enlightenment Intensive masters training.

Yoga, meditation, and self-inquiry are vehicles designed to carry a person all the way to what Berner described as the doorless and windowless "Temple of Truth." But to get inside the temple, a person needs to step entirely outside of the mind, momentarily leaving their thought-based identity behind. Anyone wanting to experience this shift must pass through what Berner called a "discontinuity." It is this discontinuity that separates our ordinary mind-bound consciousness from enlightened awareness. No mechanical practice or formulaic technique can bring this shift about, as willful efforts only further engage the mind. All a person can do is intend to directly experience the Self and remain open to the possibility of this quantum leap occurring. Here's a teaching of Berner he captioned Crossing the Barrier to Enlightenment:

> "When you arrive at the wall of the palace of truth, you will know that you've come up against something significant. It's not enlightenment, as there's no glow to your experience, and nothing has happened that means enough to end your search. Yet it's clear that you're up against something qualitatively different than all your previous layers of confusion and misidentification. You hit this seemingly impenetrable wall, which may also occur to you as a chasm separating you from the Truth. That chasm is only crossed by what could be called grace, a leap of faith, or good fortune. It always entails a discontinuity, a break between states with no apparent connection. Even if you've had an enlightenment experience before, getting to the next level of enlightenment is the same thing all over again. At this point, all you can do is intend to have conscious, direct knowledge of yourself as you truly are. Just intend, just be open, and either it happens or it doesn't."

These teachings brought to mind *The Cloud of Unknowing*, a Christian text written by a fourteenth century mystic who says that a human soul wanting to know God must pass through a "great-forgetting of all things temporal." According to its anonymous author, this cloud of unknowing is entered in silent contemplation, which stops thought and ushers in a period of inner darkness, sometimes called "the dark night of the soul," that is described as a necessary precursor to illumination.

Six months after the Toronto training, Lawrence was offering a five-day intensive in New Mexico. Returning home, I immediately booked flights. The training had been excellent, and I wanted Danna to meet Lawrence, but I also wanted an opportunity to apply all I had learned in my studies. A spacious home situated in a stretch of desert with no visible neighbors provided an ideal setting, and I quickly came to the place where my mind had emptied itself. Doing dyad after dyad, the abyss separating me from the Self grew palpable. On the third morning, I got up a little after three o'clock. Climbing out of my pup tent, I slowly made my way across a sandy stretch of ground, careful not to step on any of the prickly pear cactus that dotted the landscape. I was headed toward the main house, where there was room to meditate and do yoga before the first dyad started at 6:00.

I stopped to gaze up at the night sky, which was brilliant and star-strewn. Suddenly it was replaced by a vision of the universe that all these years later I can liken to an image from the James Webb space telescope. It was vast and emanating light in all directions, grand enough to dwarf the self-sense of the little me beholding it. Confronting this seeming infinitude, something became self-evident. The light radiating throughout it was not just dead photons. The whole cosmos was alive and shot-through with consciousness. With this knowing, the vision disappeared, and any remaining shreds of my skin-bound identity with it. Nothing happened externally, but the inward impact was like a simultaneous earthquake and thunderclap. The next thing I knew, I was sitting up from where I had fallen on the sandy desert floor. In that indeterminable time-out-of-time, I had glimpsed an undeniable truth. Existence is an interconnected whole permeated by direct self-knowing. While differentiated in expression, each of us in essence is that whole in its entirety.

It is not enough to hold a hypothesis, even an accurate one, in the mind. Doing only this, the truth never appears. A genuine aspirant must do vigilant soul-investigation. Before receiving direct knowledge of the divine order, there will always be what yoga calls a "false vision." The false vision may reflect real knowledge, but anything held in mind is like the image in a mirror. It is not the thing itself, and always reversed in some way. This is why an aspirant must keep one principle in mind—"I am making a journey from false knowledge to true knowledge. Until true knowledge of the highest is gained, I will not be satisfied with anything less." Absent this determination, progress is bound to stop. Direct knowledge of the divine order is different from the knowledge obtained through the study of scripture or even through contemplation. It throws light on the real meaning of everything. This knowledge comes only through samadhi, which is why it is the summit of yoga.

I was not transfigured by this experience. To the contrary, I came back to a state of consciousness entirely familiar to me, albeit one struggling to take in the enormity of what I'd just encountered. The experience was so unexpected, and occurred so quickly, that my first response was a mute question, "Did that really happen?" But there was no room for doubt. With the help of multiple intensives, I had stumbled into the temple of truth, passing through a discontinuity just as Berner had described. The dyads leading up to it had cleared my mind, and the vision ushered me to its threshold. While awe-inducing, the vision was only a mental phenomenon. It served as my entry point, but yours would be altogether different, and anyone else's different still. After dusting myself off, I continued to the house and sat in meditation, passing in and out of a state of beyond-mind awareness previously unknown to me.

> Charles Berner on Samadhi and Self-Inquiry: "Samadhi is beyond the mind and senses. It's impossible to adequately describe. But it may be helpful to know that it is through samadhi that you come to know directly that what you are, and what God or the Ultimate is, are the same. Your own divine nature comes into union with God or Truth. On the way to samadhi, a depth process of self-inquiry will naturally occur in your meditation to take you beyond the mind.
>
> At some point in this process, the mind goes through something that reminds me of a scene from an old movie I once saw. A bunch of kids were sitting in this unhitched covered wagon. One of them accidentally released the brake, and the wagon started rolling down a hill. Some mothers noticed and began running after it. They weren't fast enough, so the men hopped on their horses and gave chase, but the wagon kept going faster and faster. Everybody was shouting, screaming and panicking. The action got louder and wilder. And then the

wagon went off a cliff. As it flew through the air, there was a sudden silence.

A similar thing happens to the mind. It gets busier and busier. It reaches a frantic pitch. Finally, it goes fffsssssst and there is a moment of complete ego annihilation. This moment of de-identifying from something that only moments ago you were convinced that you were feels like death. But to have an enlightenment experience, you must pass through this discontinuity, this break in identification and consciousness. It's common to want to turn and run at this point. You don't want to bring about the death of that which you are accustomed to thinking of yourself as being. Mastering intensives, I've had many people cry out, "It's not my ego that is dying, it's me! Don't you understand?" This feeling of terror is a tremendous barrier. But there is always this gap in enlightenment work, this void between the unenlightened and enlightened states, this timeless instant in which you cease to exist. In truth, the process of crossing it is not dangerous. You go through the same barrier every time you fall asleep and wake up. If I were to reassure you that you did the same thing just this morning, you might reply, "I didn't do that; it just happened by itself." Which would lead me to say: That's the way this is going to happen too, but you have to be open to it."

The remaining two days of dyads provided me with time to integrate my experience and explore operating from this new perspective. I had no delusions of being able to live in this state—it was just too big—but a chasm had been crossed. After stumbling inside the temple of truth, I had been able to re-enter it in meditation, and enlightened awareness no longer felt off limits to me. When the retreat ended, I could honestly say that the question What am I? had been answered. But I was left with a new inquiry: How could I act to solidify my truth-knowing and allow it to infuse my life?

Arriving home from New Mexico, I knew the right way forward for me was not signing up for another Enlightenment Intensive. The ones

I'd done had delivered their promised breakthrough. Instead, I needed to find a way to reliably access that level of consciousness, using the glimpse provided me to extend my meditation practice into the realm of samadhi. And that felt possible because I had a visceral, experiential sense of where the path of yoga was leading.

> *As long as the stage of meditation continues, the thought stream continues and the mind veils the soul. When meditation is raised up one step – when it takes the form of samadhi –thoughts dissipate. Eventually the mind becomes no-mind and the soul can be realized. It should be remembered that the self-change registered in such a realization is not in the soul. The soul exists as always, but it's now known. This reveals an important principle. Only when the activity of the mental faculty ceases can the soul be known directly.*

BE A DISCERNING STUDENT

The path of yogic meditation is meant to continue after an initial experience of samadhi. Dharana and dhyana, which up to now have been the mainstay of meditation, become precursors for the trifold practice of samyama. The samadhi needed to commence samyama practice is one step beneath the level sought in the Enlightenment Intensive. It's the ability to access, even if momentarily, the pure, object-less consciousness underlying the mind, as explained in the next chapter.

Anyone having what the Enlightenment Intensive calls "a direct experience of truth" will find their memory of it a curious one. They will be able to recount the story surrounding it—much like I have done here—but the experience itself is a different matter. Ineffable yet indelible, it is unlike any other memory held in the mind. What remains continues to reverberate as a living reality. To recollect it is to return there, if only for a millisecond.

APPLYING THIS CHAPTER IN PRACTICE

The ability of a question to direct the mind is astounding. Imagine that you are working on a complicated project in your office. Spreadsheets and papers cover your desk. You are fully occupied in concentrated thought. Suddenly, a visitor cracks opens your door and asks, "Sorry to interrupt, but where is the nearest bathroom?" Instantly, you are able to set everything aside and answer, "Go down the hallway through the double doors and the ladies' room is on the right." The woman thanks you, and you return to your focused work. But in that brief interim, when her question was hanging in the air, you had to entirely clear your mind.

Yoga uses the questions posed in self-inquiry to interrupt our habitual mental patterns and direct attention to the task of self-knowing. This enables us to cut through mental clutter and begin working through all the surface notions of who we are that block access to the deeper layers of our being. Every attempt at self-inquiry pokes a hole in the mind-based identity. Through repeated efforts, the shell of our surface persona becomes porous. If subjected to a sustained effort, it is destined to crumble and reveal something surprising and unexpected. That doesn't mean the work is quick or easy. Swami Kripalu conveyed that in a colorful way by likening the process of self-inquiry to *chewing on a steel garbanzo bean*.

Looking back, the importance of the Enlightenment Intensive in my spiritual life cannot be overstated. The series of intensives I took opened a doorway into a dimension that would otherwise have remain off limits. Opening that door admittedly required some degree of forcing. I would never have been able to inquire deeply enough to crack SK's proverbial steel garbanzo bean without the Intensive's contemplation technique, structured round-the-clock schedule of dyads, and group support. Absent the catalyst of the Enlightenment Intensive, it's likely I would have continued my mind-based meditation indefinitely, and the next few chapters would remain unwritten.

Although Self-realization (atman vijnana) can be gained by either samyama (yogic meditation) or atman-vichara (self-inquiry), it is only made thorough (embodied) by applying it in life.

CHAPTER 17

YOUR HIDDEN CAPACITY FOR SUPERCONSCIOUSNESS

The samadhi for which you are practicing is called with-seed samadhi. It is a superconscious state (atimanasa) in which mentation ceases but the seed of mind continues to exist. After meditation ends, the seed sprouts and all your mental tendencies again take shape, but rid of some contradiction or lower quality. There is a second samadhi in which the purified mind is absorbed into the Absolute. Before mastering the first, this second without-seed samadhi cannot be known.

Although the Sanskrit word *samadhi* is standard vocabulary for contemporary yogis, it is seldom discussed in practical terms. Most teachers rarely mention it, considering it a far-off or even unattainable state. In contrast, Swami Kripalu spoke openly and encouragingly about samadhi. My interest was piqued every time I ran into a reference. While still a novice practitioner, the things he said left me motivated to pursue it, even though I felt my chances of ever advancing to that stage of yoga were slim.

Sage Gheranda says, "None is so fortunate as one who attains samadhi." Having inspired us, he continues, "There can be no yoga without samadhi." In this second statement, a critical doctrine is laid down. Only through samadhi can the fluctuations of the mind be stopped. Absent this, there is no possibility of realizing absolute truth. While yoga calls this ability to know beyond mind samadhi, it matters little what name is used as long as meditation proceeds to the point in which the mind is directed towards its supporting source, yielding direct spiritual knowledge. Sage Gheranda concludes by saying that samadhi is unattainable without the grace of a guru. Only a lit candle can light an unlit candle. This need to be instructed by a realized person cannot be negated simply because some people do not agree with it. In these brief statements, Sage Gheranda has given us an invaluable teaching.

Twenty years passed before the Enlightenment Intensive sparked an inflection point in my spiritual life. Igniting it was the intensive's technique of self-inquiry. Responding again and again to the directive, "Tell me what you are," it became apparent that I could not be any concept, image, belief, or narrative storyline held in my mind, as the true self stands apart from what yoga calls "the mental instrument," able to examine its contents. Encountering this level of my being beneath and beyond all the mind's conditioning, there was no going back—it was impossible to un-know.

That's when Swami Kripalu's teachings on samadhi became relevant to me. Studying them, a deep yearning arose to move past the boundaries of my mind-based meditation. Like a snake itching to shed an old skin, I felt driven to slough off my burdensome egocentric identity, or at least the most troubling aspects of it. To start actually doing that on my cushion, I needed to learn how to shift from dhyana into the beyond-mind state I now knew was possible. An undertaking of that magnitude requires trustworthy guidance. Interpreting SK's samadhi teachings in the light of his life story, it became apparent how deeply he was steeped in the subject.

Not long after starting my earnest practice, no sooner would meditation begin than I would forget my physical existence. This was my initiation into samadhi. Patanjali says that progress in samadhi depends on the effort made – whether mild, medium, or intense—with the highest samadhi coming quickly to those practicing intensively. Other sages explain the pace of a student's progress based on the caliber of grace received from their guru. Given my divine teacher and energetic practice, I fully expected to complete my samadhi in six months. One year passed, then two years passed, with me eagerly awaiting the highest samadhi. Ten years passed, with samadhi looking deeper still. In that condition, the pain of separation is so great that day and night become one. Today, twenty-seven years have passed, but no more am I impatient. I enjoy my sadhana, and that is why I continue doing it. Having surrendered to the Lord, I do not care whether my practice completes in this or some other lifetime.

For three decades, SK strove to summit the mountain peak of samadhi by patiently ascending all its ridges and lower stages. Seeing this sequence modeled in his life offered real insight, as it helped me drop my naïve fantasy of leapfrogging into some ultimate state that would magically resolve all my problems. To follow the path he blazed, my next step was to focus on those teachings targeted on entering and moving through the stages of what yoga calls *sabija* or *with-seed* samadhi. Gaining this clarity of purpose, I saw that life could not have provided me with a better mentor.

Samadhi is a continual concentration by means of which all external objects, and even one's own individuality, are forgotten. The truth of One Being makes its appearance in the state of with-seed samadhi, even though various thoughts continue to pass through the mind. Yogic aspirants must understand that the pilgrimage of samadhi is long. With the advent of samadhi, an aspirant begins to move in and out of the superconscious state. After distractedness ceases, absorption ensues, and the pure consciousness behind the intellect is unveiled. The yogis believe that true Self-knowledge is sure to descend into such a mind. However, meditation must continue until the aspirant remains continually aware that they are atman and not the body-mind. Only when they recognize this as their natural state (sahaja vastha) can they rightly be called Self-realized. This is a brief description of the changes brought about by the practice of samyama and with-seed samadhi.

Because I found them so helpful, it is these foundational teachings on samadhi that are highlighted in this chapter.

WHAT IS SAMADHI?

The Sanskrit word samadhi is easily defined. Its literal translation is "to bring together completely," and that's a good starting place to gain the robust understanding of the term required to practice it. In ashram publications, samadhi was often replaced with the English rendering "unity consciousness," which is a good pointer at its overall yogic meaning.[1] But that's a description of its mature expression. Samadhi initially presents in quickly passing moments of undividedness whose significance is easy to miss.

The consciousness signified by the word samadhi is not an improved version of the familiar and fragmented mentalized awareness with which we habitually live our lives. Swami Kripalu described samadhi as a *superconscious state*, but that English translation of the Sanskrit term *atimanasa* is cumbersome and must be correctly understood.[2] In everyday usage, the word super means "possessing a quality to an extraordinary degree." For example, the comic book character Superman has extraordinary strength, x-ray vision, and radar-like hearing. If samadhi is conceptualized as a greatly-amplified mind, it will undermine your yoga practice, because no one can measure up to the standard of a superhero.

Fortunately, this is not what he meant by *superconscious*. The Latin word super originally meant "over and above" or "operating at a higher level." Interpreted correctly, superconscious means "the highest and most fundamental level of our consciousness." Anthropology can help clarify what yoga is trying to point out. The earliest known species of humans are classified as homo sapiens or "the one who is aware." They

[1] As referenced earlier, pioneering neuroscientists Andrew Newberg and Eugene d'Aquili in studying contemplative practitioners describe the highest meditative state with a term that tracks closely with the yogic definition of samadhi: Absolute Unitary Being.

[2] SK was not alone in teaching Westerners that samadhi is a superconscious state. Swami Vivekananda appears to have been the first yogi to use that term, which appears in his 1896 articulation of Raja Yoga. Decades later in the 1920s, it factored prominently in the Kriya Yoga of Swami Paramahansa Yogananda, who founded Self-Realization Fellowship. In the 1960s, it was adopted by Swami Rami, the founder of the Himalayan Institute, who taught a method he called *Superconscious Meditation*. The word is often traced back to William Walker Atkinson (1862-1932), an American occultist and pioneer in the New Thought movement, who used it to refer to a level of the psyche that he believed was in a superior position to the unconscious, subconscious, and conscious levels of mind commonly recognized by psychology.

are called the clever hominids because their intelligence is displayed in sophisticated tool making and all sorts of complex behaviors and survival strategies.

Modern humans come later and are classified as homo sapiens sapiens or "the one who is aware of being aware." Scientifically speaking, it is this metacognitive ability to reflect on our own existence and the experience of being conscious that distinguishes modern humans. Along with adaptive value, it makes an entirely new domain of endeavors possible that includes literature, philosophy, science, and the evolution of culture. A cadre of renowned thinkers argue that it is this capacity for self-reflection that makes us uniquely human. Many mystics and yogis believe that this same ability, when developed to its full potential, is what equips us for Self-realization.

This is the superconscious state described by SK in his teachings on sabija samadhi, which in meditation can be thought of as an overarching "awareness that is aware of itself." While inconspicuous and easy to overlook, this background awareness is always available to us. It remains clear and undivided, and is never fragmented, even when the foreground thinking mind is cluttered, conflicted, or confused.

Sage Patanjali says in the Yoga Sutra that sublimating the activity of the mind is samadhi. Sage Vyasa explains in his commentary that samadhi is a thoughtless and superconscious state. A person who faints enters a thoughtless state. How is that different from samadhi? A person who has fainted is simply devoid of thought, while a yogi in samadhi remains completely conscious of their thoughtless mind. It is this second stage of awareness the sages called the super-mind (atimaṇasa). A fainter does not attain wisdom, bliss, or salvation. But all these are gained by a yogi who activates the superconscious mind and masters samadhi.

THE SUBJECT-OBJECT DICHOTOMY

Philosophers have analyzed human experience for millennia, and their disciplined terminology can point out the hiding place of your capacity for samadhi with great precision. A basic premise of philosophy is that all experience requires a subject and object. A subject is a person or more specifically a "conscious entity." An object is something that can be perceived by a subject. This includes external objects like a book or tree. But it also refers to internal objects, such as a sensation in the body, a feeling in the emotional system, or a thought in the mind. Understanding this premise, any philosopher will immediately grasp why all the mind-based stages of yogic meditation (dharana and the various levels of dhyana) make use of an object of contemplation to steady the mental faculty, sharpen attention, and fine tune the meditator's subjective experience.

But technically-speaking, samadhi does not occur in the realm of experience. Philosophy is completely correct in asserting that all experience takes place in the mind and requires a subject and object. Samadhi occurs outside the mind and off its perceptual screen of objects, whether gross, subtle, or very subtle. In Swami Kripalu's way of thinking, samadhi occurs in the soul. In philosophical terms, samadhi is a shift into the unalloyed subjectivity prior to subject/object consciousness. This is where the capacity for samadhi is hiding in you—in the silent space of self-knowing before the arising of what yoga calls the "I-thought."

The Hatha Yoga Pradipika tells us that a yogi seated in samadhi is not conscious of sights, sounds, touch, tastes, or smells. Nor does he differentiate between himself and others. His mind is not sleeping, nor is it awake to the outside world, because he has gone beyond all experience to the place where truth may favor us.

Philosophy is an intellectual discipline. Its tools are designed to explore the outer limits of the mind, but no further. The task of going beyond the mind is a confounding one, even for gifted mystics and accomplished yogis. That's because the mind cannot be transcended by volitional acts or willful practices, which only generate more experience and further stir the mind up in the process. Nor does the beyond-mind state result from simply ceasing action and allowing thoughts to settle. Inaction may slow down the mind's spin cycle, but subconscious impressions will continually surface to keep it oscillating. But if the attention of a focused mind is raised to its highest expression as pure objectless consciousness, and held there, the mind's connection to its animating source is cut. In response, it will grow silent and still. This pause in the mind's activity is the opening to samadhi.

After practicing various yoga techniques, the body ceases to be restless and the mind becomes steady. As outer and inner activity slows, the aspirant approaches samadhi. At this point, knowing what to do with the mind is indispensable. The sixth chapter of The Bhagavad Gita guides us: "Whenever the mind roams or wanders, it should again and again be held in the soul." A well-instructed aspirant of samadhi will not involve the mind in any activity other than that.

A STEP BEYOND WITNESSING

Swami Kripalu's earlier teachings detail the pivotal role that *witnessing* plays in yoga. It withers away shortcomings in the yogic process of character building.[3] It helps you to step back from the outer-directed senses to experience pratyahara—Chapter 13. And once a critical mass of concentration has been generated in dharana, witnessing resumes to enable you to pass through all the subtle stages of metacognition that comprise dhyana—Chapter 15. This ability to witness the activity of the mind is equally important in all forms of therapy. Without the psychological-mindedness that witnessing brings, a client is unable to surface old hurts, discern harmful patterns, and be with the powerful emotions and sabotaging self-talk associated with them. Regardless of the means employed, only a person aided by a strong witness can do the inner work required to change the tenor of their mind.

But as you approach the stage of samadhi in your yoga practice, you must understand that the usefulness of the witness has run its course. To proceed any further, you must take what Zen monks call "the backward step" into a new domain prior to the subject/object dichotomy. Continued witnessing will only hold you back.

The Upanishads tell us how a yogi enters samadhi. "As its wood supply is exhausted, a fire is extinguished without doing anything.

[3] See Chapter 17 of *Swami Kripalu's Yoga of Success and Self-Realization.*

Similarly, as thoughts vanish, the mind automatically dissolves into its source." First you must hear this teaching. Then you must understand it. Finally, you must properly practice the techniques of yoga until mind becomes no-mind, allowing you to recognize samadhi for yourself.

Approaching samadhi, almost every spiritual seeker enters a cul-de-sac in which they expend a great deal of energy trying to enlighten the mind. It's impossible to illumine the ego, the heart-centered authentic self, or even the witnessing observer that stands silently at the end of the line of all our mind-based identities. While ardent meditation can make each of them increasingly transparent, the mind is only a reflector of spiritual light. Its nature is not luminous, or in yogic terms "self-effulgent." A single sentence culled from the Upanishads is all that's needed to distinguish these subordinate identities from the true Self and source of your being. "It alone shines."

In the practice of samadhi, the witness can be thought of as a bridge to cross over, which explains a traditional teaching that admonishes students, "Don't build your house on a bridge." If you remain entrenched in the interim position of the witnessing observer, it is likely to become the seed of what is sometimes called the spiritual ego. Identified there, you may follow all the rules and do all the practices, feeling proud of your self-discipline. Or you may fall short on both these counts and deem yourself a spiritual failure. Either way, you will not awaken beyond mind because the pure primordial consciousness we are can never be an object of mental awareness. To know the Self directly, you must cross the bridge and leave the witness behind. Freed from the witnessing perspective, the Self's shining nature grows increasingly apparent and attractive.

Samkhya philosophy tells us that to go beyond the mind is to know the Self and realize its independence from all levels of manifestation. A Samkhya student strives to discern that they are not the body, nor its actions, nor the mind or its thoughts, nor the ego (ahankara) who is having the thoughts, and not even the witnessing observer (drashtha) of all these lower levels. In the Yoga Sutra, sage Patanjali uses Samkhya philosophy to teach samadhi as the yogic means to consciously go beyond the mind and become established in Self. And what is the means of samadhi? Sage Patanjali tells us chitta vritti nirodaha, quelling the thought waves of the mind. Only one no longer possessed by distracting thoughts and these lower levels of identification can answer the question, Who am I?

REALIZATION DOES NOT RESULT FROM SAMADHI ALONE

Established in pure object-less consciousness and basking in the light of the Self is as close to realization as one can get through anything that can be practiced. While Swami Kripalu did not conflate samadhi with Self-realization, he taught that a yogi intent on practicing the samadhi of pure consciousness was not only knocking on the door but likely to enter it one way or another.

Sage Patanjali tells us that a meditating yogi established in the superconscious state attains to a purity of spirit (adhyatma prasada) that inevitably brings with it a special kind of knowledge (prajna). Lord Krishna also describes this purity of spirit gained through with-seed samadhi. He says that one set in pure intellect becomes self-controlled and finds all their sorrows coming to an end. With the ignorance of a yogi meditating in this higher consciousness steadily being dispelled, the direct knowledge that throws light on the real meaning of everything is sure to dawn.

ECHOES IN CONTEMPORARY TEACHINGS

While Swami Kripalu pointed out our potential for samadhi, there is no getting around the ponderous nature of the term superconsciousness. And my attempt to explain it through anthropology and philosophy may only compound the problem! But a survey of current teachings makes it clear that today's luminaries are using different jargon to proclaim this selfsame truth.

Much like yoga, Theravadin Buddhism is a potent force

reshaping society through its contemporary expression as the Mindfulness Movement. Mindfulness is also a bit of a gnarly term.[4] Jack Kornfield defines it as "that quality of mind which notices what is happening in the present moment with no clinging, aversion, or delusion." Jack's protégé, Tara Brach, carries this basic teaching into the realm of samadhi: "The Buddha taught that holding onto anything, including a sense of being the observer, obscures the full freedom of awareness. At those times, we might ask "Who is aware?" We might also ask, "What is aware?" or "Who am I?" or "Who is thinking?" We bring mindfulness to awareness itself. We look into awareness. By inquiring and then looking into awareness, we can cut through and dispel the deepest illusions of self that have held us separate and bound."

Eckhart Tolle experienced a spontaneous spiritual awakening at twenty-nine and spent the next few years integrating and stabilizing it.[5] In the process, he authored *The Power of Now*, which many have called a modern gospel. Eckhart offers a practical approach to conscious living that is not aligned with any religion or tradition. One idea core to his teachings is that humankind's problematic behaviors are grounded in an inability to see reality clearly because of the mind's obscuring filters, which are composed of its past-tense conditioning. He encourages students to "Realize deeply that the present moment is all you have. Make the NOW the primary focus of your life." In subsequent teachings, he promotes "The Practice of Presence" to access a samadhi-like state: "Presence arises when we free ourselves of incessant thinking and unconscious reactivity, rolling back the ego, so our essential self can

[4] The Pali word "sati" was first translated as "mindfulness" in 1881 by a British scholar named Thomas William Rhys Davids. Ever since, the aptness of that term has been a topic of debate. Davids based his translation on the Mahasatipatthana Sutta, which emphasizes the practice of sati or "watching how things come to be and how they pass away." Practiced deeply often via breath-based meditation, sati leads to a state of samadhi that transcends conventional notions of mind, an end state that arguably makes the term "mindfulness" misleading. Despite this objection often voiced by depth practitioners, mindfulness offers a good starting place for practice, and for that reason remains a central concept in Western Buddhism.

[5] Eckhart Tolle's spontaneous awakening has many parallels to that of the Indian Sage Ramana Maharshi (1879–1950), who spiritually awoke as a teenager in response to the death of his uncle, and is the inspiration behind many contemporary expressions of what is sometimes called the "direct path of Advaita Vedanta." Spontaneous awakenings do occur, but enduring ones of genuine depth are exceedingly rare. After his awakening, Ramana Maharshi spent many years in a cave doing post-awakening practice.

shine through." In a particularly direct pointer to the realized state, he says, "Ultimately, you are not a person, but a focal point where the universe is becoming conscious of itself. What an amazing miracle!"

Michael Singer was a figure in the early days of the Kripalu ashram who has recently gained national attention as an author and spiritual teacher. In his bestseller, *The Untethered Soul*, he writes, "For the deepest meditation, you must not only have the ability to focus your consciousness completely on one object, you must also have the ability to make awareness itself be that object. In the highest state, the focus of consciousness is turned back to the Self." This succinct teaching distils much of Swami Kripalu's preliminary meditation instruction and guidance on entering samadhi into two straightforward sentences.

Many contemporary teachers cite an uneducated Indian sage who had a knack for expressing profound truths in simple metaphors. Once sage Nisargadatta was asked: "When you say, "I am in the state beyond the witness," what is the experience that makes you say so? In what way does your state differ from being a witness only?" He responded: "[Yoga] is like washing printed cloth. First the design fades, then the background patterns and colors. In the end, the cloth is plain white. The personality gives way to the witness, then the witness goes, and only pure awareness remains. Awareness colored by an object of attention we call the witness. When there is also self-identification with the designs and patterning, we call that a person. When awareness is unpatterned and colorless, it is limitless and can be called the Supreme."[6]

Current sources like these have helped round out my understanding of samadhi. While saluting these luminaries, I also have to acknowledge a tendency of some contemporary teachers to encourage novice students to immediately delve into samadhi-like practices when a recognized pitfall the ashram called "premature transcendence" is known to have serious psychological downsides. Swami Kripalu felt teachings of this depth, no matter how clearly expressed or accurate, could only be effectively applied in meditation after an aspirant had progressed through a process of character building followed by the mental development catalyzed by

[6] Quotations from: *Still Forest Pool* by Jack Kornfield, page 191. *Radical Acceptance* by Tara Brock, page 313. *The Power of Now* by Eckhart Tolle, page 101, and *Eckhart Tolle: Essential Teachings Podcast. The Untethered Soul*, by Michael A. Singer, page 37. The last piece from *I Am That: Talks with Sri Nisargadatta Maharaj* is excerpted from a dialogue on page 401.

dharana and dhyana. There is an old Tibetan saying that speaks to this pitfall and bears repeating here: "Do not mistake understanding for realization, and do not mistake realization for liberation."

> *To know the Infinite reality directly and without any obscuration or veiling by the mind—this alone can be the end product of all the different types and stages of yoga. This much is real knowledge; anything else is the elaboration of words. If someone awakens the desire for this knowing, they should be encouraged according to their readiness. In India this is understood, for if everyone was immediately fit to practice the highest, there would be no need for such a thing as a spiritual path.*

NOT ONE BUT TWO SAMADHIS

Swami Kripalu stressed the role played by the two categorically different types of samadhi in the culmination of yoga.

> *Samadhi is one but it has two stages, and the difference between them is clear. In the first stage, a yogi reaches the unifying state of with-seed samadhi in meditation, but coming out of meditation duality reasserts itself. Upon entering the second without-seed samadhi, the yogi remains at all times in the superconscious state whether sitting, standing, walking, eating, speaking, or doing anything else. The reason for this difference can be explained. In the first samadhi, the mind is separated from the body, which can then glimpse the soul. In the second samadhi, the soul is separated from the mind and afterward only identifies with itself. But a practitioner should not speculate too much about states beyond their reach. It is only by passing through the many levels of with-seed samadhi that a practitioner gains entry to this second samadhi in which duality truly disappears. Some teachings say the mind dissolves into nature. Others say mind becomes no-mind and the soul merges into God. In either case, after the second samadhi, no separate meditator remains.*

Yogis like Swami Kripalu who have progressed to the second level consistently describe its occurrence as "not being the fruit of any action" and "solely the result of grace." When it does occur, without-seed samadhi is said to bring moksha or liberation, the topic of Chapter 19.

A yogi who sits steadfast in meditation can slowly render the mind thoughtless and discover superconsciousness. In this state of with-seed samadhi, the yogi experiences the undisturbed, calm, and balanced state of mind. No aspects of this state are to be condemned for it brings truth and wisdom. But only a yogi who surrenders their self into that state, desiring nothing beyond a complete purity of spirit, can hope to know the ultimate samadhi. That liberation and salvation-granting samadhi is the result of grace (anugraha) alone.

BE A DISCERNING STUDENT

The practice of a profound state of meditative absorption referred to as "samadhi" is central to both yoga and Buddhism. The historical Buddha taught samadhi as one step on his Noble Eightfold Path that is often rendered in English as "right concentration." In Buddhism, samadhi is a state of one-pointed attention practiced to develop mindfulness (sati) and verify the Four Noble Truths by gaining insight (vipassana) into the impermanence of material existence and the empty nature of self. Buddhists cultivate and value samadhi for its ability to attenuate and ultimately bring an end to suffering (nirvana). While Buddhism in general does not emphasize the various levels of samadhi as much as yoga, it recognizes they exist as differentiated states referred to as *jhanas*—see page 175—and some schools stress their practice.

Similarly, samadhi is one of Patanjali's eight limbs of yoga. Yogic samadhi is a spectrum of metacognitive states that progressively reduce mental fluctuations. The first level of samadhi is a state of steady concentration obtained through the practice of samyama that is often described as "resting in pure consciousness" that enables a meditator to observe the mind's activities. That samadhi is a precursor to a deeper meditative state in which there is no object of concentration and the unfettered mind becomes absorbed in what yoga calls "the Self." Yoga schools differ with some characterizing this state as "Divine communion" and others as "a oneness with the Absolute." Yogic samadhi's full expression is an abiding state of transcendental awareness indistinguishable from its ultimate goal of liberation or moksha. In summary, both yoga and Buddhism consider samadhi a pivotal state of consciousness, and a tool to transcend ordinary mental states and gain insight into deeper truths.

APPLYING THIS CHAPTER IN PRACTICE

When you experientially realize that samadhi is simply the shining forth of your essential nature, meditation becomes the simplest of practices as the clear light of consciousness reveals the shadowy nature of mental darkness. While only its lower expression, this samadhi is qualitatively different from the rarified but still oscillating mind states of dhyana and adds an effortless element to meditation that is intrinsically fulfilling. Although a lot may remain to stabilize this direct self-knowing, any "seeker" who enters samadhi to some extent becomes a "finder." Even when lecturing on the intricacies of yoga's highest states, Swami Kripalu retained his sense of humor as reflected in this anecdote.

When I was doing my sadhana in Malav, there was a sister who used to serve me. One day she bowed down to give me my meal, and I could see she was weeping. Feeling her distress, I asked, "My daughter, why are you crying?" Then I sat still, ignoring the food to make sure she gave a true response. I was momentarily speechless when she exclaimed, "Because I have lost my buffalo. She wandered away three days ago, and I have looked everywhere but not been able to find her." Taking in what she said, I recognized this was a serious matter. In India, a buffalo costs six or seven hundred rupees. For a villager like this sister, that is a lot. Wanting to make her laugh, I said, "I will go in samadhi and try to see where your buffalo is." Samadhi is for finding God. I don't think anyone can go into samadhi and find a buffalo. But I said this without thinking. It did make her laugh, which led me to also laugh. Another sister overhearing our conversation surprised us both by saying, "Since Swami is laughing, you will definitely find your buffalo." This story does not reflect well on me. A yogi has to be careful in what he says and never attach his name to any miracle. The honest way is the only way. But God is a big comedian, and by next morning that sister found her buffalo. God worked the miracle in a way that gave me the credit.

CHAPTER 18

SAMADHI IN PRACTICE

Distraction vanishes when meditation yields a moment in which the light of pure consciousness is seen. Such stray glimpses generate rays of hope that it may be possible to reach your goal of Self-knowing. Strictly speaking, a glimpse is not samadhi. Yet it is not incorrect to consider it an immature samadhi provided the inspiration gained is used to attain to your meditation's mature and steady state.

Samadhi is often thought of as an end-of-the-road experience of adept yogis. While this view may suffice for a novice asana student, it will impede the progress of anyone who becomes a regular meditator. As soon as contemplative practice begins, it is important to look at dharana, dhyana, and samadhi as an integrated whole. In his book *Science of Meditation*, Swami Kripalu explains that it's only by utilizing all three of these together that substantial progress can be made:

A yogi established in self-reflective meditation enters a state of pure consciousness. In that state, the thinking mind (manas) is freed from its misconceptions and the intuitive mind (buddhi) holds only truth. To reach to that high degree of mental purity, Sage Patanjali advises a yogi to combine dharana, dhyana, and samadhi into a single practice called samyama (bound together disciplines). Indeed, it is through this trio of concentration, meditation, and samadhi that anyone so desiring can succeed in making the mind one-pointed and advance toward the true goal of directly knowing the reality beyond it. Mastery in meditation unfolds slowly and is not accomplished all at once. An infant grows into a child, and childhood gradually gives way to adulthood. In the same way, dharana grows into dhyana, and over time dhyana matures into with-seed samadhi. Practiced together, these three are the trustworthy means to the end stages of yoga.

Efforts to restrain the thinking mind are front and center while learning dharana, but the nature of an externalized mind is to wander, and even a disciplined effort will bring only a modicum of success. More progress can be made as the thought stream begins to flow smoothly in the introverted state of dhyana, which considerably lessens the mental effort needed to remain present and focused. But even in deeply absorbed states of mind-based meditation, the thought current is continually shifting. It is only when the pure awareness underlying the mind is recognized that it becomes possible to steady the attention in the sustained way signified by the term samyama. A meditator who gains this ability to rest—even momentarily—in object-less consciousness has reached an important milestone in yogic meditation.

Even a fledgling meditator can lay the foundation for samyama practice by leaving a few minutes at the end of meditation to let go of all technique and relax into this essential awareness. Once this template is understood, you can begin to divide your meditation time into three roughly-equivalent intervals. In the first, breathe your way into meditation and use your object of contemplation to establish a steady focus (dharana). In the second, allow yourself to relax and enjoy the state of flow (dhyana) that accompanies inner witnessing. It is in the final interval, when all effort ceases, that opportunities to enter samadhi will present.

In the tumult of daily life, our awareness inevitably gets tangled up or "blended" with the parade of thoughts, feelings, and sense perceptions passing through the mind. After settling into meditation, Danna and I have found inquiry an effective tool to return to the what is sometimes called the "unblended state." An overarching view of the body-mind is required to contemplate a question like "What am I?" or "What's true here?" I know that for me it was coupling the practice of dharana and dhyana with self-inquiry that opened my mind to the higher expression of meditation I was seeking. While inquiry or some other yogic tool may help get you there initially, you can eventually gain the ability to move into the pure, object-less consciousness of samadhi without any formulaic technique. More and more, meditation becomes a natural process in which the preliminary steps of dharana and dhyana position you to rest in what Swami Kripalu called the *superconscious state.*

> *Meditation is an inner journey toward the Absolute truth. Truth makes its appearance in the state known as with-seed samadhi, even though it comes and goes with various thoughts continuing to pass through the mind. It is not possible to dwell in samadhi without elevating the mind through its lower states of dharana and dhyana. Knowing this, a truth-seeker should be content to approach the summit of the highest samadhi by practicing dharana, dhyana, and with-seed samadhi for many years. The mental peace born of this contented samyama practice is the only means available to hasten progress.*

SHARING MY EXPERIENCE

Swami Kripalu was a private person. Despite that predilection, he spoke openly about his yoga experiences when doing so might assist other practitioners. Everything generic I want to convey about samadhi has already been said. To go further, I have to share personally about my efforts to progress from the composite practice of samyama into deeper levels of samadhi, not to claim any special status, but to own the potential of this path for anyone who gives themselves to its faithful practice.

After multiple Enlightenment Intensives, I found myself unable to resume my prior meditation practice. Focusing on the breath, witnessing the inner flow of feeling and thought, and praying to an external God no longer appealed. After years of fruitful engagement with these techniques, they now brought on a mild sense of revulsion. Even the pure awareness underlying the mind seemed tinged with an element of frustration.[1] All I wanted was to be one with the ultimate reality, the

[1] My antipathy for these focusing techniques was a temporary reaction. I currently use all of them in my ongoing practice, but in their proper place as rungs on the ladder of yoga. This excerpt from Charles Berner speaks to the limits of resting in content-less consciousness: "The truth is that you are not a looker, desirer, doer, or experiencer. If you can disentangle yourself from these basic points of view, you are likely to still be identified with consciousness. Arriving here, you have made a lot of progress. While on the right track, you just haven't finished the job. Yes, there is

presence of which I'd glimpsed and remained palpably real to me. But my sense of this ultimate see-sawed between opposites. Sometimes it felt like the All of Everything with which I could align myself. At other times, it was the innermost essence of my being and only true identity. Swami Kripalu must have passed through a similar period, as he clearly describes this dilemma and explains its solution.

Beginning meditators find themselves constantly distracted by the extroverted mind and senses. To overcome distraction, attention is directed to a supporting object. In this stage of dharana, a gross object provides the support needed to attain concentration. When the mind grows focused, distractions noticeably decrease and pleasant inner states arise. In this stage of dhyana, a subtle object best supports the introverted mind in remaining steady and peaceful. As the meditator approaches samadhi, the need for an object of meditation is automatically done away with. In order to move beyond the polarizing mind, meditation must center only on the Self, leaving aside all objects or other means of support to enter sabija samadhi. This is the beyond-mind meditation that leads to Self-realization, revelatory knowledge, and bliss.

Intently meditating on the Self, I had the first in a series of novel experiences. One second, I was fully present on my cushion. In the next, a dream-like image of a towering highway-paving machine filled my mind. As it crept forward, it left behind a gleaming expanse of pure black asphalt. For a moment, I was dumbfounded by this strange vision. Then its symbolism came clear. Ultimate reality is a seamless whole; there is no crack anywhere through which it can be entered. While black and devoid of light, it is also gleaming and radiant. All anyone can do is open to its all-encompassing and paradoxical nature. Receiving this message, I passed into a non-conceptual state.

Exactly what I mean by "a non-conceptual state" is difficult to convey. I was not rendered unconscious, as had happened in most of

---

this level of pure consciousness, but the true individual is not consciousness. You are the one who is capable of consciousness. Most of the journey to enlightenment is finding out who you are not. But de-identification alone is not enough. You must have conscious, direct knowing of the one who is left after all the de-identification."

my prior samadhi-like experiences. Nor did my consciousness noticeably increase. The experience—if that is the right word—was silent and devoid of mental content. Only afterward could I conjecture about what had happened. Writing today, it's tempting to say that I "merged into this" or "expanded into that" because the shift that preceded it felt significant. But the truth is much simpler. The outer world fell away while I remained acutely aware. I can't authoritatively claim this was sabija samadhi. I can only say it was altogether different from my experience of dharana and dhyana as those terms are used in the Yoga Sutra.

Sage Patanjali tells us that samadhi is citta vritti nirodha, which means a state in which the mind's modifications are restrained. The deciding factor in this sutra is the word nirodha, which I'll explain further to give you a clear and scientific understanding. The common meaning of nirodha is "restraint," and you might think that stopping a quarter of the mind's modifications, or one half, or three quarters, would all be different degrees of nirodha. That reasoning would be correct with regards to the previous stage of dhyana. But in the case of samadhi, you have to add one extra word to Patanjali's sutra. Only the complete stoppage of the mind's modifications will produce samadhi. Even if this stoppage is momentary, it will produce what yoga calls nirodha-vastha, a temporary state of cessation. This is the first samadhi, which serves as a practitioner's entry point into yoga's highest stage.

A few days later, a similar progression repeated. One second, I was wide awake on my cushion. In the next, an image appeared of a multistory house with many rooms. In each of the rooms, a different "me" was evident. In the light-filled kitchen, I was happily cooking a meal with Danna. Adjacent to the kitchen was a small and dimly lit study, where I sat working at my desk. On the second floor there was a bedroom with the door ajar where I was arguing loudly with my mother. In a little space in the attic, I sat before an altar absorbed in meditation and ignoring the rest of the household. These are only some of the multiple identities that I saw simultaneously in action. But then it became clear that the house represented the psyche, and the real me was somehow outside the house observing all of these personas. Receiving this message, I again entered a non-conceptual state.

A week or so later while meditating, I had a vision of myself having climbed most of the way up a steep alpine hill. As I kept trudging forward, I passed through one gate after another following a slalom-like path. Before stepping through the final gate, I turned to look over my shoulder, expecting to see the long trail I'd taken outlined by its sequence of gates. Bewilderment overtook me when there were no gates to be seen. Turning back toward the hilltop, the final gate I'd been standing before had vanished too. All these incremental steps were only there in my mind. Objectively, they had no real substance. Receiving this message, I again entered a non-conceptual state.

Soon after that experience came yet another with a parallel theme. Suddenly, I was standing on a high mountain ridge looking down at a jewel-like lake gleaming in the valley far below. Without thinking, I visually descended a winding footpath through the woods and quickly found myself on the bank of the lake, where a long wooden dock extended into the water. Walking to the end of the dock, I knelt down and peered into the water. Lowering my head, I could see my face mirrored in the lake's surface only inches away. Poised there, the absurdity of my current meditation practice came clear to me. Upon reaching the outer limits of my conceptual mind, I stop short of making contact with what lies beyond. Receiving this message, I tumbled headfirst into the water and entered a non-conceptual state.[2]

Modern psychology is well-acquainted with the extroverted mind but knows little about the capacities of the introverted mind. Perhaps that is why psychologists call it the unconscious. By pondering a scene or series of events, a poet or painter can bring an artistic vision before their mind's eye. But these visions of the extroverted mind are not as

[2] It would be nice to say these lessons became permanent features of my character, but I still find myself on the lookout for some connecting crack through which the mentalized me can complete the spiritual journey while remaining intact. At times, I try to pretty-up or fix some ugly facet of my personality. And whether climbing to new heights or descending into my depths, I remain a striver even while knowing the usefulness of this stance has long run its course. Like everyone, I have character flaws and personality quirks that make me cast what Carl Jung called "a shadow." Having seen and made peace with these patterns and traits, they have lost much of the power they once had to block my growth and effectiveness, but still remain operative.

impressive as those generated by the introverted mind. Water turns to ice when it reaches the required degree of coolness. In the same way, thought waves are converted into visions when the required degree of mental fixation is present. That is why a meditator who confronts a dilemma will see its solution as a vision. When they arise all of a sudden, it can feel as if some divine power is inspiring them. It is visions like this that enabled me to accomplish various stages of yoga that otherwise I would never have mastered.

At this point in my life, the remarkable creativity of the intuitive mind was known to me. But the sudden arising of these meaning-laden images in meditation, and their ability to be a portal into something seemingly non-mental, was a new phenomenon. I've since learned that psychologists are aware of these "thought-image amalgams," which occur naturally in the hypnogogic states that lead into sleep. Swami Kripalu's life story and teachings on samadhi are peppered with references to a *beyond-mind state* he encountered early in his sadhana that forcibly separated his body-mind from his soul, catapulting him into states of samadhi and non-duality (advaita). In his renunciate practice, this transition was sudden and tumultuous.

When the bodily kriyas and mudras begin, a practitioner is struck senseless and cannot imagine their final expression. Such a yogi leaves the realm of duality before the mental faculty has grown stable. The mind of a yogi who quickly crosses to the far shore of samadhi joins with the soul and becomes nothing but soul. Although this is a harbinger of victory on the path of non-dual accomplishment, a yogi experiencing these changes in a matter of months may behave like a child, an idiot, or lunatic until they can stay continually in the soul. I myself remained in this condition for a year and a half, unable to recognize samadhi from swoon.

It was clear the householder practice that had anchored my adult life was once again carrying me into unfamiliar territory. While a bit confounding, these experiences conveyed no sense of threat or overwhelm. Yet the void I was encountering felt alien enough to make me wonder, "Would my familiar identity be somehow swallowed up by this non-conceptual state making itself known to me?" All that was certain was I wanted to keep meditating.

Initiatory experiences regularly arise on the path of yogic meditation but seekers fail to recognize them. Understanding this, a seeker should remain alert to unusual experiences. By closely observing any ones that repeat, their characteristics can be identified and they can be used to progress along the right path. At first, it is easy to mistake brass for gold. But once the unique characteristics of gold are recognized, it is easy to distinguish between them. It is in this way that a seeker should test the validity of their meditation experiences by comparing them to the teachings of the great sages. Yogic meditation is a discipline to realize the gold of samadhi, but illusions also arise and over-enthusiasm often prompts a seeker to evaluate their progress in a liberal way and accept the brass of lesser attainments. Despite their apparent similarities, don't misinterpret any swoons of unconsciousness as samadhi. Instead, recognize Self-awareness as the differentiating factor between the two, and continue to practice with patience and faith until you attain the superconscious state.

MAKING SENSE OF THESE EXPERIENCES

The fireworks that accompanied these initial forays outside my known limits soon passed. Meditating in the months afterward, I found my ability to relax into this non-conceptual state growing. Gradually, I became able to abide there for periods, wakeful and alert but with relatively little mentation. Slowly it became apparent that this wasn't a mind state at all. It was a foundational level of my being that had been covered over by a cataract-like accretion of mental conditioning and thus lost to consciousness.

Reading this truncated account, you may have already connected the dots between these meditation experiences and the vision of the cosmos that knocked me to the desert floor in New Mexico. But in my life, four eventful years separated them. In part for that reason, I was blind to this link. Another reason is that the Enlightenment Intensive is an active process that builds energy and generates breakthroughs. In comparison, these solo meditation experiences were undramatic enough to occur as altogether different. But gradually the understanding dawned that I was moving through a discontinuity and touching into the same unmediated Self-awareness I'd momentarily encountered in the Intensive. As the passage through this discontinuity grew familiar, it felt increasingly self-evident that this awareness was not only foundational to my psyche, but somehow core to reality itself.

Looking back on these experiences, I can see how each countered an ingrained mental pattern that was blocking my practice. When the first occurred, I was spending a chunk of my meditation time looking around for some hidden passageway to the ultimate. The seamless asphalt let me know that there is no such crack to be found. The second revealed that my attempts to unify all my different self-expressions was similarly misguided. My true identity is neither an ideal version of my disparate selves, nor a combination of all my roles and responsibilities. It is something else that exists outside the bounds of the conceptual mind. To this day, the third experience makes me laugh at myself. I am such a striver, clawing my way up the spiritual path through one self-created gate after another to reach some imagined summit. But any idea of progressing along a path to a future enlightenment is a misnomer, as no series of incremental steps to get you inside the Temple of Truth can be pinpointed. The fourth experience reinforced the same message in terms of descending into the depths of my being. It gave me the best single piece of realization instruction I've ever received. When it comes to touching into the unconditioned reality that lies beyond the mind, drawing close is not enough. You must be willing to get wet now.[3]

Writing today, I can't distil the effects of a dozen years of daily meditation into a simple story line. I can only share my sentiment that what's emerged from my ongoing practice occurs to me as astonishing. As I continued to meditate in the wake of these visions, this vague point of contact with a non-conceptual dimension of myself slowly matured into a rooted connection to something whole and worthy of being called "the ground of being." Resting there had the effect of kryptonite on my mind, and I came to understand Swami Kripalu's statement: *The*

[3] Meaningful symbolic images still arise fully-formed in my mind while moving into meditation. Having grown familiar with the process, it has ceased to be dramatic. Instead of anything universal, it is more likely that I am just wired in this visual away, and others would receive the inner messages they need in different formats.

beyond-mind state gives a yogi one-pointedness in the beginning, and the non-sprouting of all mental tendencies in the end.

I did not experience this rooted place as an object outside of me upon which to focus attention. It was the essential me, and so much more than me, these two realms uniting in a way that my sense of ultimate reality ceased see-sawing between opposites. As the signal emanating from this undivided place grew stronger, the noise of the mind grew less and less attractive. In that increasingly silent sanctuary, my yearning to be one with the whole could be satisfied without any loss of individuality. And as for striving, a part does not need to seek a hidden wholeness when it experiences itself as a piece of an obvious unity. Sitting each morning, my experience of this ground of being steadily took on the quality of love.

The controversial but insightful spiritual teacher Bhagwan Shree Rajneesh said there are two types of spiritual seekers. The first are contemplatives who find love through meditation. The second are romantics who find meditation through love. It appears I fall into the first category, as meditation has revealed that I am not just a skin-bound body-mind but a living soul in communion with a verb-like God, coinciding in love as two and one.[4] I've always related to life as a mystery that in the final analysis can't be known. While that's still true for me, my conception of what that means has changed. It now occurs to me that existence is a bottomless mystery that can be infinitely known in layer after layer of divine revelation. As these layers unfold, the relationship between me and the larger reality grows richer and more love-filled, leaving me buoyed by a consistent feeling that my cup is overflowing.

I make no claims to my experience passing the scriptural tests for with-seed samadhi. All I can really say is that my post Enlightenment Intensive meditation practice has enabled the spiritual drive that has dominated my life to slot into what currently feels like its right expression. I am certain there are deeper levels into which I can and hopefully will unfold. But having found a way to offer my devotion and bask in a sense of grace that consecrates the moment, I'm content in the knowing that anything more must come from drinking deeply of what's before me now, both on my cushion and in my life.

[4] As an artist and poet, Danna falls into the second of Rajneesh's categories. Her yoga and meditation has taken her on a different yet parallel journey. Much like myself, she has grown content to rest in what she calls "the love field" and trust what unfolds from there. The fact that SK's teachings have brought two very different individuals to a similar stage of meditation suggests there is something universal in their efficacy.

Yoga is not prudish in characterizing the pure but dualistic love that is the hallmark of sabija samadhi when experienced theistically, and that distinguishes it from its final nondual expression. Neither was Swami Kripalu:

Everyone knows that it's through sexual intercourse that new life is born. Yoga calls this coming together of a man and woman sambhoga, which means "pleasure conjunction." Yogis also know that there is a state of samadhi called samyoga, which means "yogic conjunction." This joy-bringing state of the mental faculty is not the final samadhi in which mind no longer exists. It is only the beginning of samadhi—the entrance permit that opens a passage to the unscalable top rung of the ladder of yoga. By means of this initial samadhi, joy erupts from the void, and it is seen that there is no difference between the living soul, the love-filled God, and the universe. This is why the Bhagavad Gita tells us that it is only through a devotional conjunction with divinity that divinity can be attained.

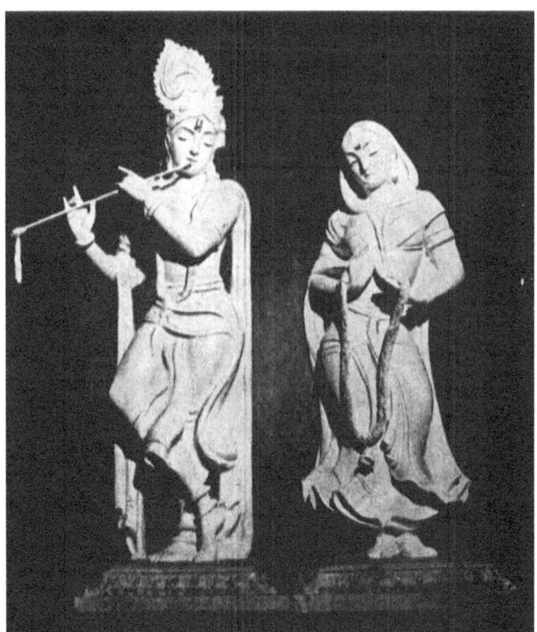

Meditating after these experiences, I have come to see the symbolism of the first of two murtis or sacred images that SK kept on his altar as a sculptural representation of the yogic state of sabija samadhi or divine communion. Radha is the Divine Feminine and embodied soul that longs to reconnect with its spiritual source. Krishna is the Divine Masculine and cosmic soul whose flute plays the love song that calls the embodied soul back to God consciousness. Reunited, they dance in ecstasy.

SHOULD I TRUST MY EXPERIENCE?

Swami Kripalu taught that a yogi practicing with-seed samadhi will go on to display certain characteristics received as *a gift from the highest soul.* First is *para vairagya*, a total detachment from the ups and downs of life, which brings with it a loss of all fear. Next is *ritambhara prajna*, a special kind of intuitive knowledge that he defines as *direct knowledge of the divine order.* Then come all eight of the yogic powers or *siddhis.*[5] Of course, none of these yogic attainments bore any relationship to my practice, which caused me to doubt that I'd made any progress at all.

The first chapter of The Yoga Darshana is titled "Samadhi." Its forty-seventh line says that a yogi who becomes thought-free for a long time gains direct knowledge of the divine order. In that state of omniscience, the mind does not exist, and such a yogi is without ego. His faculty of discrimination enables him to fluently explain scriptures he has never before heard. He has penultimate detachment, and thus no fear. Consequently, his pain and delusion disappear, and he is always serene. While possessing miraculous powers, he has no desire to exhibit them. These are the signs displayed by one who ascends to the thought-free level.

Fortunately, I happened upon the teachings of Roy Eugene Davis (1931-2019), an American yogi and disciple of Paramahansa Yogananda who also emphasizes the importance of learning how to meditate in the superconscious state. Davis says a yogi meditating superconsciously will discover intuitive knowledge unfolding in a three-step realization process. First a meditator discerns that "the essence of my being is pure consciousness." Next comes the insight that "my essence is not different from the essence of Ultimate Reality, which is also the essence of all other beings." He says the final step cannot be conveyed in words but

[5] *Ritam* means *truth; bhara* means *full of*; and prajna means *direct knowing.* Yoga defines ritambhara prajna broadly as intuitive knowledge arising from meditation. SK used this term narrowly to make the point that realization is not gained through resting in pure consciousness alone, which is the initial level of samadhi practiced in samyama. Realization only results when one's practice of samadhi bestows a special kind of knowledge. *Para vairagya* translates as *supreme non-attachment.* The ashta or eight yogic siddhis are detailed in the Yoga Sutra.

describes it generally as "a shift in perspective" that "occurs through grace." Davis's more-relatable teachings are entirely consonant with those of Swami Kripalu.

Studying Davis's teachings, I had to admit that coupling self-inquiry and yogic meditation has brought me a subjective knowing that I can't objectively verify, yet feels undeniable. Through it, I've seen how a single intelligence and energetic source sustains me and everything else in the universe. This is where words break down, as I've not seen this with my eyes, or through any kind of inner vision. Just as SK teaches, I've come to know it in moments when the mind's activity subsides and only the simplicity of this oneness remains. It's not that I don't forget and forego this knowing—as I do, every single day—but it's become a truth I can return to, and one that grows ever more self-evident as I continue to practice.

With-seed samadhi is also known as wisdom-bringing samadhi because through it one attains doubtless and true spiritual knowledge. Ordinary knowledge may be forgotten, but this special knowledge born of samadhi is not forgotten even in difficult circumstances. The Gita describes such a yogi as "having seen the equivalence." Verse 6:29 tells us: "One who is possessed of yoga sees his soul in all beings, and all beings in his soul." Verse 5:18 adds: "With the same evenness of love they behold a Brahman who is learned and holy, a cow, an elephant, or a dog, and even the man who eats a dog." Some texts call this knowledge of the soul (atman). Others call it knowledge of the Absolute (Brahman). Regardless of name, this is the knowledge born of equal vision that is sought through with-seed samadhi.

I've not made any efforts to *master sabija samadhi* in the way that Swami Kripalu suggests below is possible. But spiritually I've become more of a finder than a seeker, and the busyness of my mind has markedly diminished. Most of my thinking is productive, and it is unusual for me to be troubled much by unwanted or intrusive thoughts, but this could certainly change in the face of a grievous diagnosis or other travail.[6] While I attribute the quieting of my mind to my yoga practice,

[6] To inject greater reality into this description of my current state, I struggle with sleep issues. I've read accounts of other meditators who describe watching their body

there is no objective way for me to say for sure. The experiment I have conducted has a sample size of one, and no control group. Your journey into yogic meditation and samadhi will undoubtedly be different, but I hope this sharing of my experience proves in some way helpful.

It is through mastering the practice of samyama that a yogi's mind passes through various superconscious states to attain sabija samadhi. Even though this first samadhi is considered very important for the knowledge of atman it bestows, it must also be mastered before the highest samadhi can arise in which the mind dissolves into the Cosmic Self. Seen this way, the first samadhi is like a seed buried in the soil during the rainy season that shoots up abruptly, and the omniscience of the second samadhi is like the tree that slowly takes shape as all the lower stages of samadhi are mastered and the yogi's self-surrender (atmanivedana) is perfected.

BE A DISCERNING STUDENT

Yoga's inclusive approach to spiritual awakening is often described by the credo: Many paths, one goal. Hearing this catchy phrase, it's easy to imagine samadhi as the shared goal integrating all of yoga's diverse expressions into a coherent tradition. In actuality, there is considerable disagreement among the major yoga schools on the nature and practice of samadhi. Each propounds its distinctive and often contradictory teachings. Scholars highlight these discrepancies as significant points of doctrinal conflict. Some go further to suggest that samadhi is best seen as a mythical notion versus any state of consciousness that objectively exists.

While researching this chapter, I happened upon a website that

---

fall and remain asleep while retaining a restful samadhi-like consciousness. As far as I can tell, SK never claimed such an ability and instead spoke of sleeping soundly through the night. Despite best efforts, I often find myself wide awake at 3:00 a.m. after a restful period of non-REM sleep. Sometimes I manage to fall back asleep. Other times I get up and meditate for an hour, after which I usually can return to bed and restart the sleep cycle. Fairly often, this results in vivid or lucid dreams that prove meaningful. While open to these issues resolving in unexpected ways, I would prefer the simple ability to dream the night away. Sleep issues are one of the known "adverse effects of meditation," for more on this see the work of Willoughby Britton, PhD.

advertises itself as listing fifty-one traditional definitions of samadhi.[7] At first, I laughed. But checking it out, I was impressed by the author's diligence and rigor. Perhaps to alert students to all these differences, Swami Kripalu delineated the views of the major yoga schools on samadhi as reflected in their authoritative texts. See Appendix 5, which compiles these teachings into a brief history of the term samadhi.

Most people are not yoga practitioners. Yet social scientists know that a sizeable percentage of the population reports having had one or more "peak" or "mystical" experience. Personal accounts suggest some of these experiences correspond to high yogic states including the lower stages of samadhi. In my estimation, what converts these serendipitous moments of non-ordinary consciousness into a transformed life is repeatability. To access these realms reliably, some structured approach and consonant form of spiritual practice is essential, or at least that's been my experience.

APPLYING THIS CHAPTER IN PRACTICE

Yogis and Buddhists both seek to integrate the samadhi state experienced in formal meditation into daily life. Buddhism emphasizes the practice of mindfulness and equanimity in everyday activities to cultivate wisdom and compassion. Yoga emphasizes surrender to a power greater than ourselves and the intuitively-guided actions that come from embodying the principles of karma yoga. Both share a vision in which samadhi is not a compartmentalized practice but a quality of awareness that permeates and infuses one's life.

Some yoga teachers believe that samadhi should be considered to have occurred only after its unequalled expression is gained. There is truth in this viewpoint as the end sought by samadhi is a complete dissolution of mind. As long as a student accepts that a true mastery of samadhi takes many years, I am of the opinion that samadhi's lower expressions should be recognized. This makes it more likely that subtle meditation experiences that occasionally happen by grace will not vanish but occur again and again.

---

[7] www.wisdomlib.org/definition/samadhi

CHAPTER 19

LIBERATION IN LIFE AND DEATH

Moksha is the soul's release from all forms of misery, struggle, and suffering. Only this knowledge-filled state of everlasting peace and bliss can rightly be called liberation. In the final analysis, yoga is a discipline for accomplishing moksha.

The idea of a liberation from the limits of the human condition is core to yoga and the scholastic field of soteriology, which studies the world's religious doctrines of spiritual emancipation. While moksha is the generic name for this concept in yoga, other terms are used including *mukti* (released from bonds), *kaivalya* (isolation of the soul from its entanglement with matter), and *apavargaḥ* (having moved beyond the constraints of material existence). Buddhism adopted and is now closely associated with another traditional yogic term *nirvana* (to extinguish the insatiable craving for impermanent things that lies at the root of suffering).[1] Yoga affirms moksha as a positive state on par with the salvation of mystical Christianity. It holds that once the instinctual passions are recognized as adaptive and moderated through disciplined practice, they can be sublimated into an evolutionary drive for Self-realization that when fully met satisfies the soul.

In our secular times, a student must ask if all these depictions of a *summum bonum*[2] are vestiges of earlier religious ages marked by idealistic thinking. As is true with samadhi, scholars point to a noteworthy lack

[1] Nirvana literally means to "blow out." It is an ancient yogic word that pre-dates Buddhism and also appears in Hindu, Jain, and Sikh texts.
[2] Summum bonum is Latin for "the highest good or ultimate goal," a Roman phrase for a moksha-like ideal that factored prominently in the philosophy of the ancient Greeks.

of consensus among the major yoga schools on the nature of moksha. Many text references are philosophically compelling but lack substance and often define moksha by saying what it is not. Others explain away this deficiency by saying the state exceeds the boundaries of mind-based cognition and is thus ineffable. Still others seem to mix fact and fancy, like this excerpt from the Mrgendra Tantra Yogapada:

> If the yogi practices samadhi correctly, visualizing no iconic form, and thinking nothing, he soon experiences the unfolding of his own nature as an all-encompassing vision and action, full of bliss and eternal. Once this has been attained, he is never again touched by the suffering that permeates the pernicious condition of transmigratory existence. Through the practice of this yoga, he roams the realms of his choice in his sense-free body, resplendent with all the divine perfections. Then, when the moment comes, he puts aside even this yogic body and dwells only in his own identity, a substrate of miraculous action. (Sections 61c – 63b and 66.)

These critiques should not be brushed aside, as the differences they highlight go to the heart of the teaching. For example, some yoga systems declare that liberation is only possible with the death of the material body. Others are adamant that a truly liberated yogi is endowed with an immaterial and immortal body. Among the theistic schools, moksha is variously defined as merging into the deity, becoming identical in essence to the deity while remaining an individuated soul, joyously accepting one's proper role of divine servitude, or even rising to a status of incarnate omnipotence superior to the unmanifest deity. In non-theistic systems, the self might be preserved in liberation as in Samkhya, dissolved away forever as in Advaita Vedanta, or was never there to begin with as in Buddhism. While cognizant of all these incongruities, Swami Kripalu was among the faithful, one-pointedly pursuing moksha into his final days:

I am a believer in salvation and have not practiced yoga for twenty-two years to obtain any of its lesser accomplishments. Yet the path of moksha is long, and the formidable difficulties encountered on it only become known after embarking. I consider myself fortunate to simply stand in line with all those seeking liberation. The greatest lights of this world have advanced to this stage of total liberation. Only such an elevated soul can bestow a competent liberation teaching. Not understanding the subtleties, we call these great souls spiritual masters and think of them as authoring texts. In truth, the scriptures they left behind are of divine origin, written down by these obedient souls as all-merciful God acted through them to keep the path of liberation open to humanity.

HOW CAN I GET TO MOKSHA?

Soon after Swami Kripalu arrived in America, he gave a short talk that ended with time for questions and answers. The first question was posed by an ashram resident eager to reach the apex of yoga: "How can I get to moksha?" Swami Kripalu's answer helps us not lose sight of his basic teaching that both self-actualization and Self-realization are prerequisites to liberation practice.

Moksha is the goal of saints and accomplished yogis. The path to moksha cannot be tread by an ordinary person, who must first walk the path of dharma, which is open to everyone. On the path of dharma, one becomes a virtuous and skillful person able to exercise self-restraint. Then yoga techniques can be practiced to awaken the heart and illumine the mind. Unless you have successfully passed through these preliminary stages of yoga, it would be misleading for me to tell you that moksha is the path to God, everlasting peace, and freedom from all suffering. The idea of moksha should not be used to escape life. If you become a great and successful person, and still feel a desire to be liberated, then the path of moksha will open to you.

MOKSHA FOLLOWS SAMADHI

In all the meditation-oriented schools of yoga, liberation is pursued through the ardent practice of samadhi. Swami Kripalu affirms this principle: *While the ultimate goal of yoga is moksha, a yogi attains this only after freeing himself completely from the bonds of the body and mind through the practice of samadhi.* Yet he also emphasized that *moksha is solely the result of grace.* Confronting this dichotomy, I've come to believe that his personal experience was that samadhi is by itself a necessary but insufficient practice. To lead to liberation, meditative samadhi must be accompanied by a humble and heartfelt surrender to a power greater than ourselves.

Imagine yourself standing on the bank of a river so wide that it clearly cannot be swum across. The pursuit of moksha is like this—as it soon becomes obvious that liberation cannot be gained without taking the help of the boat. We may think the boat is our indomitable courage, unwavering faith in the guidance of our guru, trust in the accuracy of yogic scriptures, or the direct knowledge gained in samadhi. It is true that each of these is needed. We must be bold and keep studying and practicing until the opposite shore is reached. But the boat is grace.

LIBERATION BY CASTING OFF THE BODY

Many Vedic texts depict yoga as a means to exit the body and liberate the soul. This view gained momentum in the Upanishadic era when groups of spiritual strivers (sramanas) appeared in northern India seeking to escape what they saw as an endless karma-driven cycle of birth, suffering, and death. Among these sramanas were yogic sages, Buddhist monks, and Jain ascetics. All these systems depict liberation as something that can only happen when the soul is freed from the constraints of the physical body. This idea is exemplified in the historical Buddha, who was recognized as having attained nirvana during his lifetime but only obtained his ultimate release (pari-nirvana) in death. It is also reflected in the Yoga Sutra, which says "a yogi able to control the nerve currents gains the coveted ability to leave the body at will." (3:40) The same idea appears in the Bhagavad Gita in a devotional form:

> Hear now of what the Vedic seers call the path to the eternal, which can be reached by those who live the holy

> life and strive for perfection. If when a person leaves their earthly body, they are in the silence of yoga, and closing the doors of the soul, they keep the mind in the heart, and place in the head the breath of life. And remembering me (God in the form of Krishna), they utter Om, the name of the eternal (Brahman), they traverse this path supreme. Those who in the devotion of yoga rest all their soul ever on me, very soon come unto me. And when those great spirits are in me, the abode of joy supreme, they never again return to this world of human sorrow. For all the worlds pass away, even the heavenly realm of the gods. They pass away and return. But those who come unto me go no more from death to death. (Verses 8:11-16)

Swami Kripalu acknowledged this form of liberation called *videha mukti* or "liberation by casting off the body."

There are two kinds of liberation: the first occurring as the body is cast away (videha mukti) and the second obtained while living (jivan mukti). Teaching lineages place importance on one or the other. A yogi doing sadhana for a long, long time reaches a point where all karmic action is completed. No attachments or motivation to take any action remain, even those that maintain the life of the body. It is like a person ending a long journey. On reaching their destination, there is no place left to go. When the mind of a yogi has been emptied of all desires in this way, it becomes the cause and condition of their liberation. Entering the intimately joined realm (the samadhi of divine union), an indescribable type of bliss is born and the body is easily dropped. I am not yet at this stage, but my sole remaining desire is to attain liberation in life (jivan mukti), or to leave this body remembering the name of God (videha mukti).

Today, the work of many hospice professionals is guided by their understanding of the dying process as an opportunity to consciously transition into the after-death state. In the initial psychological phase of this process, a person is compelled to move through the stages of denial, anger, bargaining, depression, and acceptance identified by the Swiss psychiatrist, Elisabeth Kubler-Ross, as they come to terms with their terminal condition. As the body loses its ability to sustain life, the nervous system falters, the egocentric mind unravels, and the subtle connections that anchor the soul on the physical plane dissolve. Leaving the body, the soul is often said to enter a tunnel of light through which it can move onto its next expression.[3] Yogic texts add the idea that a spiritually awake individual can recognize what is happening and enter the liberated state as the dying process completes.

The following teaching story titled "Grandfather Wants Pancakes!" suggests that a householder yogi can die in a way consonant with the ideal of Videha mukti.

Once there was an old grandfather named Manubhai. He was quiet and good natured. Each evening Manubhai retired early, which enabled him to get up early to do his spiritual practices before anyone else awoke. Long widowed, the whole family held him dear. One morning, the household was abruptly awakened an hour before the sun had arisen. Grandfather was banging his hands loudly on the kitchen table and shouting, "I want pancakes." No one knew what to think. Their quiet grandfather always ate khichari (a traditional mixture of rice and lentils) for breakfast. When they entered the kitchen, they saw that grandfather was not disturbed but glowing and blissful. After many years of devoted sadhana, grandfather had realized the truth that morning. Coming out of meditation, he noticed that he was very hungry. Grandfather said nothing to explain himself, yet everyone sensed that something pivotal had happened and were happy to make him breakfast. Grandfather lived in this state for several years. When his time came, he departed this world in peace.

---

[3] Modern views on death and dying can often be traced back to the teachings of Tibetan Buddhism and the *Bardo Thodol*, a text used by monks to help people navigate the dying process. While commonly called *The Tibetan Book of the Dead*, many of its central concepts are derived from earlier Buddhist, Upanishadic, and Vedic thought. The seminal work of Elizabeth Kubler Ross is detailed in her bestselling book *On Death and Dying*.

LIVING LIBERATION

Moksha isn't a word that has much currency in today's yoga world. When discussed, it is generally imagined to be a lot like the state of the glowing grandfather depicted above. After attaining enlightenment, grandfather lives untroubled by the push-pull of the mind. When he reaches the end of his natural life, he is able to peacefully transition to whatever is next. As a lineage holder in the Pashupat yoga tradition, Swami Kripalu's conception of moksha was radically different. He subscribed to a Tantric view that came to fruition a thousand years after the Upanishads and proclaimed that a yogi need not die to attain the liberated state. By practicing its brand of hatha yoga, a truly liberated yogi is endowed with an immortal body.

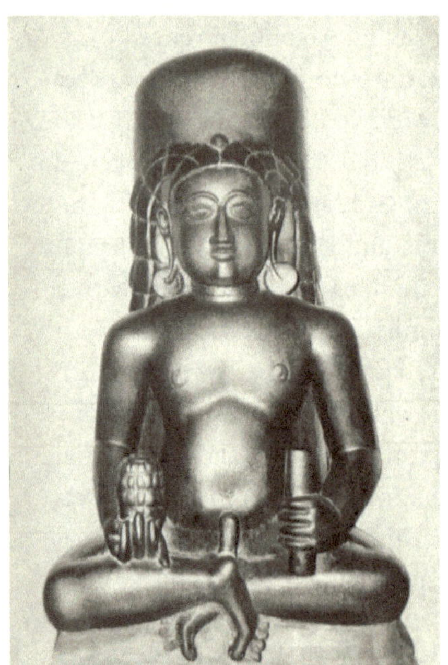

This is the second *murti* or *sacred image* that SK kept on his altar, which is a sculptural representation of the highest yogic state of nirbija samadhi or divine union. The Shiva lingham symbolizes the unmanifest Absolute devoid of any attributes. The yogi Lakulish is fused to the lingham to convey there is no separation or difference between the liberated yogi and the Absolute itself. This suggests that all of us, knowingly or unknowingly, are faces on the Absolute.

The masters of Tantra consider freedom-while-still-alive to be the ideal state. They say, "The yogi who is set free in life through obtaining the without-old-age-and-death body is the one who is really accomplished." It is because they place importance on living liberation that they teach the complete path of yoga despite it being full of countless difficulties and dangers. Through this yoga, the ordinary body is purified by the fire of a fully-awakened kundalini and transformed into a divine body. Without the presence of a few liberated-while-alive masters, yoga would become a blind tradition, and the paths of both dharma and moksha would be lost. My teacher (Lakulish) was such a yogi, so I follow the teachings of these great masters.[4]

APPLYING THIS CHAPTER IN PRACTICE

The goal of obtaining a deathless body through the practice of hatha yoga never felt relevant to Danna or me. But the idea of dying consciously has always mattered to us, and increasingly so as we grow older. That desire is reflected in the evolving set of self-created prayers that each of us inwardly repeats as we move into meditation. Danna sometimes expresses her last wish this way: "And when it comes my time to die, may I let go into the Infinite without a backward glance." Along with prayer, I have explored how the concept of liberation applies to meditation practice, whether in life or at the time of death, and the following shortlist of aphorisms distils the teachings of the Yoga Sutra into a succinct statement of its approach to moksha.

When a yogi becomes established in samadhi, the mind becomes steady and luminous. (1.47)

As the mind reflects the pure, unchanging consciousness of the atman, Self-realization becomes possible. (4:22)

The experiential wisdom (ritambhara prajna) gained in that state is filled with truth and insight. (1.48)

Beholding the distinction between the mind and Self (atman), false identification ends. The mind inclines toward the Absolute and begins to long for liberation (kaivalya). (4.25-6)

When all other aims or attachments cease to hold any interest, the

[4] The mind-bending story of how a skeptical and scientifically-minded Swami Kripalu came to accept the reality of the divine body is detailed in the fifth chapter of *Dharma Then Moksha.*

yogi enters that samadhi (dharma mega samadhi) which brings an abundance of virtues like a rain-bearing cloud. (4.29)

In that samadhi, all afflictions, hindrances, and karmas are overcome. (4.30)

Then the substrate of the oscillating mind, having fulfilled its purpose, dissolves, enabling the Self to abide in its true nature. (4.32 and 1.3)

It is in this way that the supreme state of liberation (kaivalya) manifests. (4.34)

Swami Kripalu was not one to entice students to pursue pie-in-the-sky spiritual goals. Looking at his teachings as a whole, he rarely spoke about moksha. In its place, he emphasized two defining words of the Maha Upanishad, *Vasudhaiva Kutumbakam*, which together mean *the whole world is one family.*[5] He sang the praises of this maxim for reflecting *the highest spiritual realization*. This was his approach to a practical form of liberation that anyone can apply in their life.

The highest principle of Sanatana Dharma is Vasudeva Kutumbakam, which guides us to continually develop the feeling that the entire world is our family. Householders practice this at home by making sacrifices for the happiness of their loved ones. Business people give of their time and resources to better their communities. Noble saints move through society affectionately inspiring good character, principled thinking, self-control, spiritual practice, and benevolent service to those in need. As humane individuals, it is not right to think that we are free. We are responsible for our family, community, nation, and world. One who can digest this principle that we are all brothers and sisters is sure to become an embodiment of compassionate love and service. Only such an individual can truly be considered a yogi, one who has surrendered his

[5] The complete verse reads, "This is mine, that is yours, such is the calculation of narrow-minded individuals. For the noble-hearted, the entire world is one family."

life to the path of becoming a liberated being, and may rightly be recognized as one regardless of the country in which they were born.

If you were to ask Swami Kripalu how this goal of global unity and shared responsibility is to be attained, his answer would almost surely consist of a single four-letter word.

Truly the wise proclaim that love is the only path, love is the only God, and love is the only scripture. Impress this verse upon your memory and chant it constantly if you wish to realize your dreams of growth. Love is the worldwide religion. Whether the scripture you hold in your hand is the Vedas, the Bible, or the Koran, it is trivial without love. Although the Lord is the personification of love, we seldom allow Him to enter the temple of our hearts. This failure makes it difficult for us to practice true religion. Without love in our heart, its light is not kindled in our body, our home, or in our world. Love is the all-seeing divine eye and the wish-fulfilling touchstone. Love is God's only envoy, everyone's well-wisher, and the only guide on the true path. The path of love is very ancient. When I was born, I received the initiation of love. Now, with the same love, I initiate everyone else. Countless times, I have dipped into the world's highest scriptures, and I have received only love from them. Love is my only path. Lord Love is everything to me. I am, in fact, a pilgrim on the path of love. Victory to the path of love!

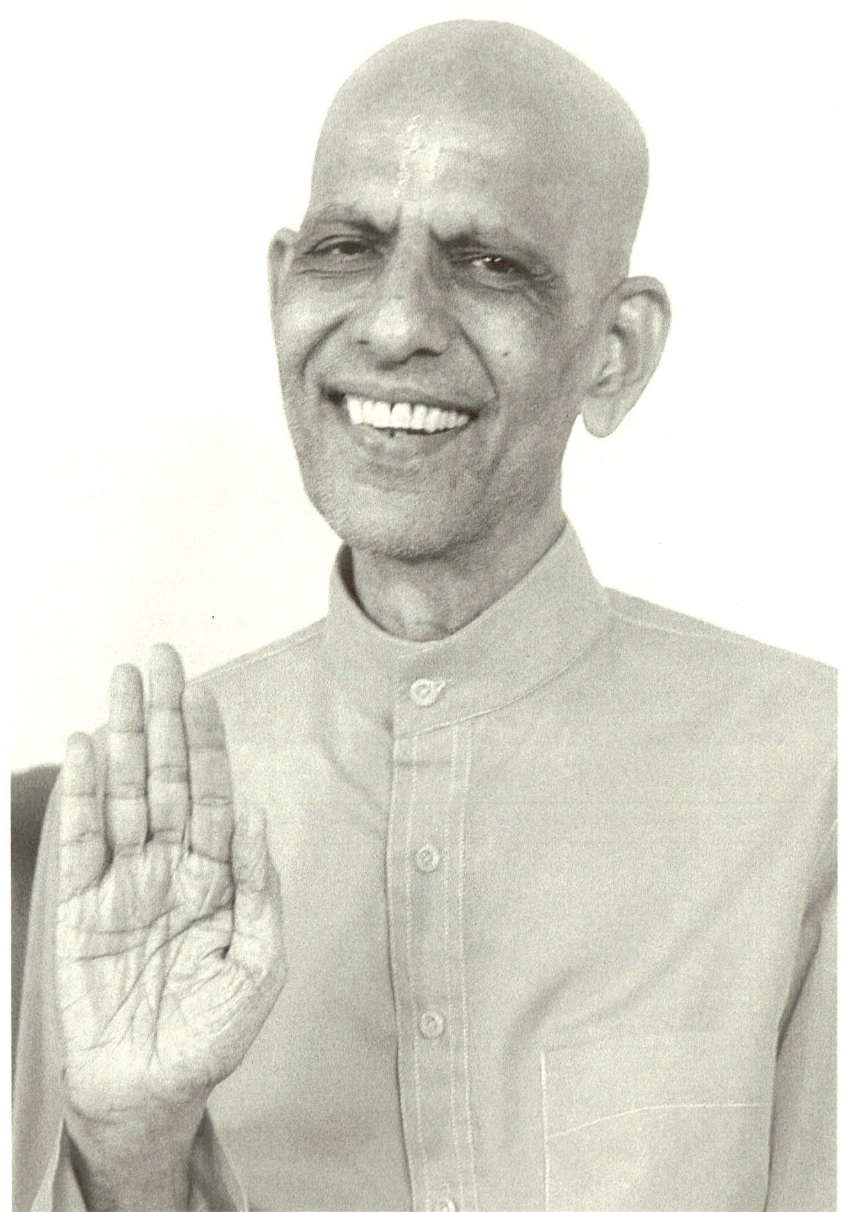

SK in blessing pose during the years he lived at the Pennsylvania ashram.

EPILOGUE

The yogic scriptures say the Divine Self residing in the temple of one's own body is the guru of all gurus. That one alone is the true teacher, and all other gurus are mere agents. Yet many great yogis have praised these agents, and even considered them equivalent to God. There is a difference between God and a fully-realized guru, and yet in another way there is no such difference.

Indian culture venerates its spiritual teachers to a degree that confounds most Westerners. Take the Guru Stotram[1], which is an integral part of the daily prayers recited by devout Hindus, and boldly proclaims: "Guru is the creator. Guru is the sustainer. Guru is the transformer. Verily, the Guru is the supreme God almighty. To that auspicious Guru, I reverently bow." This excerpt from the Siva Samhita affirms the same message but includes additional elements targeted to yoga practitioners:

> Now I shall teach you how to succeed quickly in yoga. Disciples who know this do not fail. Wisdom that comes from the mouth of the guru is potent. If not, it is barren and only brings suffering. The guru is father. The guru is mother. The guru is God. Of this there is no doubt. That disciple who zealously makes his guru happy quickly gains the reward of his teachings. For this reason, disciples should serve the guru with their actions, thoughts, and words. Everything that is good for the

[1] The Guru Stotram (Ode to the Guru) is fourteen-verses of the Guru Gita, a lengthy hymn that attributes all sorts of supernatural powers to the guru. It contains the above prayer, which is often chanted: Gurur-brahma gurur-vishnuh. Gurur-devo maheswarah. Guruh-sakshat parabrahma. Tasmai sri gurave namah. The Guru Gita is part of the much-longer *Skanda Purana*, attributed to sage Vyasa. The above excerpt from the Siva Samhita appears at 3.10-21.

> self is obtained through guru's grace, so the guru is to be served constantly or else no good will happen.

In the face of such accolades, it is easy to think that a yogic guru like Swami Kripalu must be all-knowing and possessed of miraculous powers. After scrutinizing his life and teachings, I can report that he was not a perfect person. He had shortcomings, and arguably a few blind spots. A psychoanalyst studying his biography might conclude that his zealousness in yoga arose from a cascading childhood trauma that combined with a few irrational beliefs to form a tragic flaw.[2] But having shortcomings, blind spots, and tragic flaws—isn't that true for all of us?

The record bears equal witness to Swami Kripalu's physical vitality, noble character, emotional warmth, and intellectual brilliance. He chose to channel these gifts in a spiritual direction, and together they endowed him with an indomitable spirit to not only embark upon the path of yoga but endeavor to complete it. When I met him near the end of his life, his pencil-thin, sixty-nine-year-old body emanated a bristling energy field unlike anything I've experienced before or since. Things happened in his presence that still mystify me and many others. Yet after studying his views and teachings, I'm certain he'd say that all these potentials exist in every one of us, at least in seed form.

SK never hid his faults. But he also did not closet away his highest aspirations. Perhaps the greatest gift I've received from him is the willingness to own and accentuate my positive qualities, and affirm the virtues of others, without having to deny or close my eyes to the rest. Given

[2] Swami Kripalu's father died unexpectedly when he was seven, plunging his family into poverty and at times homelessness. See Chapter 1 of *Dharma Then Moksha*. At the onset of my last book, I noted that every system seeking to guide a student's growth and development has deficits and problem areas, and promised to offer some critiques of SK's approach after its thorough presentation. Forty-five years after his death, SK's scientific views are outdated and the sexual norms, gender roles, and views on celibacy he promotes are questionable. At times, the combination of his intellectual acuity and extreme dislike of the religious hypocrisy prevalent in the Indian culture of his day expresses in teachings that can sound harsh and judgmental. His public support of the traditional guru/disciple relationship, although nuanced, could be seen to have contributed to the pattern of student abuse that became prevalent in the West, and many years later led to the dissolution of our ashram. It might be argued that I have downplayed or omitted these and other elements of his legacy. Rather than a historical account, my task has been to preserve the best of his teachings. One of his guiding principles in studying growth methods is to make use of what is good and helpful, and let go of the rest. That is what I have done here.

the fate of so many Eastern spiritual teachers who came to the West, it's noteworthy that he never fell prey to the scandals that seem to predictably arise when too much trust and power is placed in an authority figure. Part of what I believe protected him was his healthy perspective on the role of a yoga teacher.

What does a lit candle pass to an unlit candle? Only a flame that is beyond both. Does this mean that the first candle is the master of the second? Of course not. Yet it is natural for the second candle to feel a sense of gratitude, and attribute greatness to the first candle for the part played in its illumination. But the first candle has no concern for this. Its duty is simply to pass on the light. It knows that it was lit by some other candle and is similarly indebted. This is why a truly realized yogi does not possess a feeling of superiority and instead finds equality in everybody. Such persons are givers and do not want your property, or to share in your fame, or benefit from your service. It is enough for them that you want to remove the obstacles blocking you from Self-knowledge.

He was also protected by the gratitude he felt for all the students and devotees who supported him during his early years as an itinerant orator, and especially those who housed and fed him during his last four decades of reclusive practice.

I have many innocent pupils who from our first meeting believed me to be their guru and spiritual father. All my students have loved me deeply and made the utmost effort to obey my instructions, not for a few weeks but over many years. They have taken the greatest care of my body, feeding me milk instead of water, clothing me in silk instead of cotton, and even providing me with velvet seats to sit upon. I have unbounded love for these generous souls, who have been ever ready to satisfy my wishes. It is concern for them that helps me remain vigilant in my conduct to ensure that my defects do not permeate into them. Whether near or far, I never forget them, and remain constantly aware that my yogic observances have only been possible because of their service.

As someone treading Swami Kripalu's path of yoga without the benefit of much personal guidance, I paid close attention to his descriptions of how to be a good student. Alongside guru's grace, he emphasized the role of independent thinking and self-effort.

The most praiseworthy of my disciples do not blindly accept my teachings. When I tell them something, they remain objective and neither accept nor reject it. Instead, they apply what I have suggested in an experiment. In yoga sadhana or life, this is the approach that leads to true understanding. A disciple must be very honest with their guru. At times they may argue with their guru, not in an intellectual battle of wills to prove their opinion, but to ascertain the truth. It is in this way that a guru can play a great role in your growth. While it is natural for disciples to want to live nearby their guru, I have always preferred for them to reside elsewhere and do their sadhana independently. This requires them to be self-reliant. Staying near me, their individuality will not develop fully. By making proper visits, I can provide them with whatever guidance is needed. A newly-initiated disciple will never like hearing this. But their understanding will come in the future, when through their own efforts they reach the higher stages of sadhana.

Franklin Albert Jones was a controversial American guru better known by the spiritual name Adi Da. Jones was outspoken in his belief that a personal relationship with a realized teacher was required to activate the spiritual process. He challenged students like me who adopt the teachings of a renowned but deceased sage and practice them from a safe distance in a famous statement: "Dead gurus can't kick ass." There is truth in this perspective, but life left me little choice. Swami Kripalu died a few months after I met him. Later, I came into contact with a multitude of teachers, and learned a great deal from them, but none felt compelling enough to emulate. At the heart of the yoga lineage and sangha[3] into which I felt called were a dead guru's teachings.

[3] A sangha is a spiritual community that forms around a defining path or system of practice.

***

I've never hesitated to share my experience of meeting Swami Kripalu and detailing what transpired in those few hours that shifted the trajectory of my life. The full story appears in the preface to *Dharma Then Moksha*. But I never included events from earlier that day, concerned they might detract from the more important things that occurred in Swami Kripalu's presence.

As instructed, I arrived at the Kripalu Yoga ashram in time for lunch. Exiting the parking lot, I followed a stream of people up a gravel road and directly into a serving line of folding tables heaped with what I instantly recognized as hippie food. I'd been told the mid-day meal cost $5. I looked around to find a cashier to pay, and then just anyone who might be in charge. Seeing nobody fitting either description, I took my place in line. A huge bowl of salad greens was followed by an equally oversized kettle of barley vegetable soup. Then came the main dish: a warming pan stacked with lentil burgers next to a huge basket of freshly baked whole wheat rolls. Just the sight and smell of all this vegetarian food made me feel at home. There was an outdoor eating area with chairs and tables, but they were all taken. So I carried my tray to a grassy spot with a tree trunk to lean against. I didn't know a soul, but that didn't seem to matter as the scene felt welcoming. The food was darn good, and I relished it while surveying the scene.

I returned my tray and started toward an outbuilding that had caught my attention with its banging screen door. While eating, I'd noticed some women coming from there to replenish the line. I walked through the door into a rustic kitchen, where one of the cooks cheerfully accepted my five-dollar bill. I exited with some time to kill, as Swami Kripalu wasn't scheduled to appear until 3:00. I decided to stroll the grounds and was looking around to get my bearings when a middle-aged woman wearing a white sari approached me.

Smiling as if she knew me, the woman handed me a hardcover book titled *Science of Meditation*, resting on top of a folded bath towel. "If you take this path, it leads to a pond. You might want to read a little, take a swim, and then get cleaned up for darshan." Darshan was the word everyone used for the gathering with Swami Kripalu, which I'd come to understand meant "being in the presence of the guru." She continued,

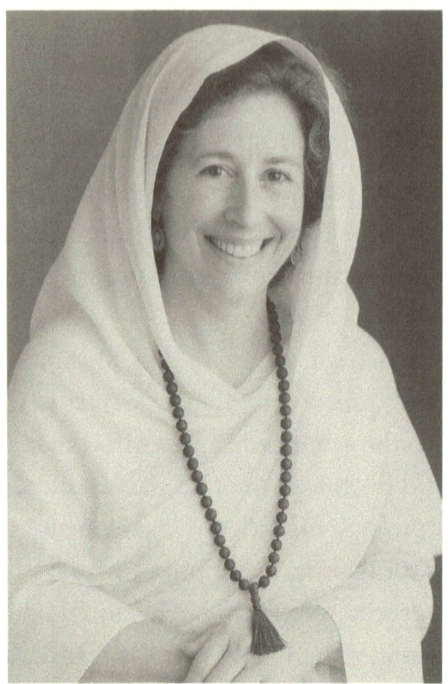

Years later I learned this woman was Frances Mellen or Ramadevi, who along with her husband Peter were early ashram leaders. Both Jonathan Foust and I clearly recall an apparently lost photo of her in a sari. This is our attempt to recreate it using Jonathan's photography skills and a little AI wizardry. Any reader wanting to experience the actual zeitgeist of those days is encouraged to watch the Path of Love video, which was created by Frances and Peter. youtube.com/watch?v=mUSCww7-XIQ

"We have a cabin you'll see from the pond. You can leave the book and towel there. Be sure to get to the chapel early. There will be lots of people, and you don't want to be late." Smiling again warmly, she turned and left.

This was decidedly not a normal social interaction, but I'd been to a few communes before and thought to myself, "Maybe this is how things work around here?" Anyway, her suggestions appealed to me, and I started down the path she'd pointed out to do just what she said. I've always been a sucker for spiritual books. Sitting by the pond, I was taken by this one. It was unusual, more a scholarly treatise on yoga than the hip counterculture paperbacks I was used to reading. I made it a point to buy a copy before leaving so I could study it closely. The pond was small, but the water looked clean. No one was around, so I shed my clothes and took a swim. Drying off and getting dressed, I spotted the cabin and began walking up a little hill to return the book and towel.

Here's where the story goes off the rails, but I can only recount what happened next. I approached the cabin and found the front door wide open and no one in sight. The place looked newly built, and I admired its neat construction, with an open floor plan and well-organized loft. Standing at the door, I saw a bath tub filled with water that was hot and steaming. I replayed what the woman had told me. "Take a swim, and then get cleaned up." It seems totally outrageous now, but at the time the only thought in my mind was, "This must be for me." I shed my clothes a second time and climbed right in the tub. In my defense, I can only say the ashram atmosphere in those early years was permeated by a palpable energy of love and acceptance. It was not unusual for a newcomer like me to become entrained in it to humorous effect.

After my relaxing bath and shampoo, it was time to head to the chapel. On the way there, I ran into the sari-clad woman again and was totally unselfconscious in meeting her gaze. I told her that I'd left the book and towel in the cabin, and she handed me a little bouquet of wild flowers. "You'll want to have something to give the guru." "Thank you for everything," I replied, and headed off for an afternoon that would stretch my mind to its breaking point.

Late that evening, I returned home with my own copy of Swami Kripalu's book, and the next morning began the meditation practice that would anchor my adult life. I followed his instructions carefully. Sit in a comfortable position. Close the eyes and remain quiet for a few moments to center yourself. Start with a prayer or affirmation of your choice, expressing your heartfelt intentions and aspirations. Conclude the prayer by asking for help "to meditate in the best way possible for me." Then take ten long, slow breaths to introvert the mind. After the last deep breath, surrender all effort to make anything happen, simply observing the activities of the body and mind. Meditate continuously for one hour, keeping the eyes closed, and ignoring external noises and distractions. When the hour has passed, come out of meditation gradually, allowing the mind time to become extroverted and reestablish control over the body.

Before coming to the ashram, I'd practiced zazen and been taught by a roshi to count my breaths. SK's approach felt a whole order of magnitude bigger. And it was so simple: get centered, offer up a prayer, breathe deeply, and let go. I'd also studied yoga in college but was ignorant of the Hindu rituals that customarily accompany a student's entry into a teaching lineage. Only years later would I reflect back on that day and realize that it had all the elements of a traditional initiation ceremony. The purifying swim and bath, an audience with the guru, a gift of flowers placed at his feet. Of course, SK knew nothing of this. He was long past accepting new disciples, and silently engaged me as he did everyone else that day. Yet there is no denying that in those minutes, something happened inside of me that resulted in my becoming his student. Even now it makes me wonder, "What is the nature of this life, which at a pivotal moment can create something so right, yet absolutely unplanned and unscripted?"

Looking back, I can trace the journey upon which his teachings and the daily practice of meditation has taken me. I can't report that all the advanced techniques of yoga arose spontaneously from the energetic power of my breathwork and meditation practice, as they apparently did for Swami Kripalu. Much to the contrary, I had to learn and apply everything outlined in this book. But all these efforts were undergirded by a deep sense of surrender to a universal power greater than my mind. As I slowly moved through the stages of yogic meditation, there were many times when I needed the help of some teaching or technique to overcome a hurdle or jumpstart my stalled progress. Whenever this occurred, the help always arrived in some form or another. A book, a serendipitous conversation, and not infrequently a sudden understanding of a SK teaching that I'd only partially grasped before. I credit daily yoga, pranayama, and meditation for keeping my antenna up and my intuition turned on, enabling me to sense whatever next step was mine to take.

In the particular approach to yoga that I teach, a practitioner surrenders to the spiritual Source from which the body and mind receives their energy. In the final analysis, this is the essence of all my teachings. It is worth understanding surrender, which yoga variously calls sharanagati or surrendering to, pranipat or bowing before, and prapatti or the giving over of one's ego.

After I am done here, I will get up and take my seat in a car. Having surrendered to the car, I can trust it to carry me forward to my desired destination. It is the same with the destination that you want to reach in the spiritual life. Does this mean that after mentally deciding to surrender to the Source you will not have to do any karmas (actions)? No, in this approach you must not only take your seat on the meditation cushion but continually deepen your capacity to perform surrendered actions. Along with keeping your thoughts and conduct pure, you may find other practices such as prayer, devotional chanting, postures, pranayama, studying scriptures, charitable service, and self-observation to be helpful. These can be done over and above your meditative surrender.

Some teachers say that only surrendering one's entire

life—including all of one's possessions—to the guru can rightly be called surrender. Does this mean that a householder has no possibility of doing surrender yoga? No, this is not true. If you are a householder, you can also practice this sadhana in accordance with your circumstances.

Even if you surrender yourself completely and boldly proceed from there, your mind will continue to be visited by fears. At times it will grow depressed. Despite steadily performing yogic activities, you will watch their results with a sense of doubt. Only after a long time does a yogi realize that all these events are occurring in order to fulfil some specific but still unknown purpose. As your observation in this regard becomes more refined, you will also see yourself grow in faith and trust. As a result, your surrender will deepen, and your soul will travel onward towards the highest samadhi.

The idea that it's possible to establish one's self in a steady state of unity consciousness lies at the heart of the yoga tradition. Frankly, I do not know if this is humanly possible. I've certainly not accomplished it. From what I can tell, Swami Kripalu never claimed to have done so. As a Kripalu Center staff member, I've been privileged to interact with many of today's spiritual luminaries. Without a doubt, I've found them awake souls and kindred spirits who found their way to some version of the same teachings and truths that have meant so much to me. By walking the paths that called to them, their lives were transformed by moments of revelatory knowing. Some have managed to persist in that knowing and keep alive its afterglow. None of them, however, have struck me as living in a steady state of enlightenment.

While I can't in good faith lure you to practice yoga with the promise of an ultimate attainment, I can say that practicing in the manner outlined in this book has taught me how to reliably tap into the power of my spiritual source. Drinking daily from that wellspring has fueled a life that's left me grateful and fulfilled. And even now and well into my seventh decade, I am still growing like a garden weed. While I've done my best to introduce you to Swami Kripalu's teachings, and explain the why's and how's of the practices he recommended, the truth is that yoga carries you deeper and deeper into a bottomless mystery. It's a lot like my experience with the woman in the sari: how could she possibly have known what I needed and provided it for me? Yet, somehow or other, yoga does work. Practiced regularly, it will deliver the goods. Or at least it has proven itself to me. You will need to do your own experiment.

ACKNOWLEDGMENTS

The renunciate mindset I donned in my youth impacted more than my yoga practice. It led me to view my life as an all-out quest for God-realization and enlightenment. The intensity with which I held that purpose drove me to leave other things behind, including high school friends, college friends, graduate school friends, and a succession of work colleagues too. Topping the list of those I'd like to acknowledge in this book that sings the praises of the householder path is anyone once close to me who feels I inexplicably disappeared on them. Despite my neglect, I've not forgotten you.

No one makes the spiritual journey alone. Along the way, a multitude of individuals, and all manner of formal and informal groups, have carried me along. It would be impossible to name any of them without leaving significant people and important role-players out. To everyone who has supported me, practiced and explored with me, contributed to me, believed in me, or simply put up with me, please receive my heartfelt acknowledgment and thanks.

Truth be told, it's always seemed I was chasing after windmills. As a result, I never expected to get very far on the path of yoga. But I always studied and practiced with a secret hope. Anything I learned or experienced along the way, I tried to understand at a depth that would enable me to pass it on should an opportunity present. That intention lies behind this book, all my other books, and every talk given, program taught, or workshop delivered. If only my efforts could shed a bit of light on someone else's your journey, that would mean the world to me. This is a sentiment that leaves me wanting to appreciate you and all my readers for caring deeply about the same matters I hold dear.

I'm fortunate to still be practicing yoga and feeling reasonably spry. But recently I attended a big family reunion that included a photographer. The wizened old man staring back at me in the pictures made it clear that time was passing. None of us knows the number of our days.

Danna is seventy-three and each week at least one noteworthy member of the 1960s generation with which we both identify is reported on the news to have left their earthly body behind. That makes me want to seize this opportunity to say to everyone who has crossed my path, regardless of whether it was for a moment, a month, or a few decades, thank you!

Even after taking this broad-brush approach, it would be ill-mannered of me not to spotlight those individuals who had a direct hand in making this book as good as it could possibly be. They include Colleen Loehr, Colin Rolfe, Eric Umesh Baldwin, Jon M. Sweeney, Kevin Moose Foran, Jonathan Foust, Justin and Adele Morreale, Kacey Wilson, Lawrence Noyes, Michael Carroll, and Stephen Cope. And not to be forgotten is my writing and life partner, Danna Faulds, who helps everything I do turn out a little better.

I would also be remiss in failing to mention by name the Kripalu board members with whom I served for over a decade and who offered me the opportunity to author this grant-funded series of books: Adam Albright, Al Weis, Connie Chen, David Piver, Diane Utaski, Dorothy Cochrane, George White, Jerry Colonna, Justin Morreale, Joan Kopperel, Konda Mason, Lisette Cooper, Marcia Feurer, Marcy Balter, Maya Breuer, Maxine Grad, Michael Potts, Sarah Hancock, Steve Dinkelaker, Steven Glick, Susan Piver, and Timothy Henry.

It's only fitting to end with a special shout out to the whole host of mission-driven Kripalu Center staff members with whom I feel lucky to have served alongside. Among them are a multitude of yogis and yoginis whose personal stories are important and well-worth preserving, but not told here simply because they were not in my close circle of friends. It also includes any individuals negatively impacted by actions taken when I was in positions of leadership, or worse yet hurt by my lack of executive skill and experience, for which I am sorry. And finally, a special prayer of gratitude for Mary Lou Buck (1937-2024), a trail blazing Kripalu Yoga teacher who offered me and many former ashram residents opportunities to interact with her dynamic Charlotte NC yoga community, and whose passing I was regrettably not able to honor in person.

May the God-force at the heart of creation, from which we all arise, and to which we all shall return, keep you always soul-evolving.

APPENDIX 1

MAKING CONTEMPORARY SENSE OF TRADITIONAL PRANAYAMA

Some pranayama techniques make the life force powerful. Others help you leave outer disturbances behind and find the peaceful place within. Still others allow adept yogis to make startling shifts in consciousness by suspending the flow of breath. It's not enough to know the techniques. You also need to learn how they are meant to be useful.

A ground breaking medical study was dominating the news cycle as I started writing this appendix. Researchers monitoring the respiration of a hundred participants with high-tech gadgetry had discovered the way each person breathes is as unique as their fingerprint. To characterize a particular breathing pattern, the researchers extracted twenty-four measures from the data including overall nasal airflow, the duration of inbreaths and outbreaths, and the shifting asymmetry between nostrils. Afterward they trained a machine-learning algorithm and found these respiratory markers were an identifier equal or better than voice recognition. More importantly, the markers correlated to established wellness measures such as heart rate variability, body-mass index, and the risk factors for anxiety and depression. Buoyed by this success, the researchers are planning follow-up studies to see if other meaningful health information can be deduced from a precise set of breathing biometrics.

What explains these findings, when inhaling and exhaling occurs to us as something so natural that we do it unthinkingly? The answer is surprisingly straightforward. Each and every human brain is unique, and that one-of-a-kind brain sits at the center of a remarkably complex neurological network linking body and mind to ensure that our life-critical respiratory needs are met. As I read the researcher's description of this network, with its ties to biochemical and biomechanical receptor sites spread across our physiology, and its special set of nerves relaying information back and forth between the nose and various brain centers to control air flow through the right and left nostrils, I couldn't help but think of yoga's age-old model of the nadis and chakras.

Instruction on how to perform the traditional yogic pranayamas is readily available. Harder to come by is an understanding of the mechanisms utilized by these techniques so they can be practiced effectively today. That's the need this series of supplemental pranayama appendices aim to serve.

NASAL BREATHING

My first dose of pranayama instruction did not come from an Indian swami. It was administered by Sister Mary Joseph, a Catholic nun and grade-school teacher. One morning while sitting quietly in class, she singled me out with a loud reprimand, "Shut your trap." Fortunately, I was not the first student assailed in this manner. Despite trying hard, none of us could understand the emphasis she placed upon keeping our mouths closed. Obviously, Sister Mary Joseph was not concerned about the quality of our respiration. Keeping our lips sealed was a matter of having good social graces. Yet she was the teacher who made me aware that when it comes to breathing in and breathing out, everyone has two options, with one of them being decidedly better.

For over a century, Western medicine has looked down on the nose, deeming it an ancillary organ. Breathe through it if you can. But if not, the mouth can take its place. Many doctors continue to voice this outdated position, even after research has shown the upsides of nasal breathing are significant. Some of these benefits are obvious and proven to a degree that every yoga student should grasp. Others are less-apparent and best seen as pieces of a scientific picture that's still being painted. But even at this preliminary stage, these findings can inform a yoga practitioner's perspective on the mechanisms underlying pranayama's effectiveness.

Everyone can understand the critical role played by the nose in filtering, warming, moistening, and slowing the flow of incoming air for easier absorption by the lungs. This makes nasal breathing markedly more efficient than its mouth-based counterpart, allowing the lung's air sacs to imbibe more oxygen from each breath. Nose hairs filter out dust and larger air born particles. The lower turbinates located near the opening of the nostrils are covered by a mucus membrane with millions of tiny cilia that capture finer particles including a range of pollutants, pathogens, and allergens capable of irritating or infecting sensitive lung tissue. All the debris collected by the mucous is swept down the throat and into the stomach, where it is sterilized and eliminated by way of the intestines. A person breathing through the mouth loses this first line of immune defense against colds and respiratory viruses, making it easier for germs to invade their system.[1]

One of the reasons nose breathing exerts such a calming effect lies in a little-known molecule named nitric oxide (NO). Nitric oxide is a gas naturally produced in the nasal passages that plays a pivotal role in delivering oxygen to the cells. When we breathe through the nose, we carry nitric oxide into the lungs, where it improves pulmonary oxygen uptake. Exiting the lungs, nitric oxide molecules open blood vessels and enhance circulation throughout the body. The popular erectile dysfunction drug sildenafil, better known by its commercial name Viagra, uses nitric oxide to boost circulation to the male genitals.

Nasal breathing has been shown to boost nitric oxide levels sixfold. This helps explain research that suggests breathing through the nose sharpens mental focus and improves cognitive function, most likely by opening the blood vessels that feed the brain. The same reasoning could apply to studies suggesting that nasal breathing may help prevent high blood pressure, heart attacks, and strokes. Alongside cardiovascular health, scientists suspect that our moods, the efficiency of our digestion, the precision with which we regulate hormone and neurotransmitter levels, the strength of our immune defenses, the ability to encode and consolidate memories, and the responsiveness of our sexual function are all heavily influenced by the amount of nitric oxide in the bloodstream.

[1] These supplemental materials draw upon multiple resources including James Nestor's *New York Times* bestseller, *Breath: The New Science of a Lost Art* (Riverhead Books, 2020), which details the benefits of nasal breathing along with techniques to regain this capacity.

Nasal breathing encourages slower diaphragmatic breathing, which takes less energy and supports better lung function than the faster breath pattern produced when using the muscles of the upper chest. In moments of stress, our breathing becomes rapid and shallow—a panting-like breath taken through the mouth. This pattern reinforces the stress by generating an affective state of anxiety. Nose breathing can break this cycle by slowing and lengthening both inhalations and exhalations, reducing the number of breaths taken each minute, a breathing pattern known to generate the opposite feeling of centeredness and calm.

Nose breathing is also known to enhance sleep quality by facilitating the smooth airflow supportive of deep sleep. This reduces incidents of snoring, disrupted sleep cycles, and sleep apnea. If you regularly wake up feeling tired with a dry mouth, nocturnal mouth breathing might be the culprit. During the day, mouth breathing reduces saliva production, lowering the mouth's ability to wash away harmful bacteria and stay PH balanced. This makes a person more likely to develop gum disease, cavities, and bad breath. Night time nasal breathing is also known to prevent teeth grinding.

For all these reasons, the most important forms of yogic breathing are those that increase a practitioner's ability to take slow, smooth, and rhythmic breaths through the nose. These are the foundational pranayamas that Swami Kripalu touted as *useful for everyone*. Research suggests that they are particularly good medicine for the sixty-percent of Americans self-reporting on surveys as "mouth breathers." Contrary to what Sister Mary Joseph may have believed, mouth breathing is not a moral failure. Many children struggle with asthma, enlarged tonsils, and recurrent coughs and colds. Countless adults suffer from seasonal allergies and other forms of chronic congestion. It's easy for anyone with a frequently stuffed up nose to gradually become accustomed and eventually habituated to mouth breathing.

Yoga and medicine agree the majority of these people can regain the capacity to breathe freely through the nose.[2] Like every part of the body, the nasal cavity and its airways adjust to meet the demands placed upon them. If taken out of regular use, they will atrophy and congest.

[2] A minority have structural or other conditions that require medical help. If you encounter significant difficulty, consult a doctor and better yet an ear, nose, and throat specialist.

A person confronted by a clogged nose will feel that it is incapable of adequate airflow. When that happens, it's perfectly normal to breathe through your mouth, in the same way that mouth-breathing occurs during heavy exercise when the body needs oxygen quickly.

Mouth breathing is the state in which I came to yoga. It took a while, but practicing short periods of yogic breathing began to open things up for me. Around the same time, I was cleaning up my diet, which also helped. As my yoga practice gained momentum, mouth breathing gradually fell away. Nasal breathing just felt better. Ever since my nose was placed back in use, it has remained open and nasal breathing is something I hardly ever think about.

It's easy for me to tell you to spend a little time each day breathing in and breathing out in a very slow and smooth manner. Nothing could be simpler than sitting down to breathe steadily, bringing all your mental and sensory awareness to bear upon the flow of breath. Yet this simple practice has the capacity to restore your health, invigorate your actions, and bring great peace into your life. While easy to learn, it takes regular practice to digest all the nuances of ujjayi and dirgha pranayamas, and discipline to persevere in their practice until these benefits are yours.

THE VICTORIUS BREATH

Ujjayi is the first pranayama in yoga's curriculum of breathing exercises and the way to start realizing all the benefits nasal breathing has to offer. Don't be fooled by the technique's complete lack of any huffing or puffing. When done with focused attention, the effects of ujjayi breathing can be profound. Create an audible sound by gently constricting the back of the throat while breathing in and out through the nose. The soothing sound you are seeking to produce is often likened to ocean waves or a soft breeze. Slowly inhale and exhale, keeping the slight constriction in the throat constant to sustain a consistent sound whether breathing in or out

The biggest benefit of ujjayi pranayama is that it dramatically increases your *breath awareness*. The sound it generates is a form of biofeedback, giving you a tool to closely monitor the quality of the breath. The unbroken flow of this sound becomes your focal point, quieting mind chatter and anchoring your awareness in inner experience. It's this heightened awareness that enables you to deeply sense and begin to skillfully regulate the breath, ensuring that each breath flows smoothly and free of strain. Gain mastery in the ujjayi breath, and it becomes the building block of all the other pranayamas.

In the basic application of ujjayi pranayama, the inhalations and exhalations are kept at equal length. As the breath slows down and flows rhythmically, the mind settles into a state of restful presence. Ujjayi breathing practiced in this way closely resembles what many contemporary teachers call "coherent breathing." That technique dates back to 2001, when researchers at the University of Pavia in Italy stumbled upon a remarkable discovery. It turns out the prayers and mantras uttered by a sampling of Buddhists, Christians, Hindus, Native Americans, and Taoists all produced a near-identical rate of respiration. The breath flows in for five-and-a-half seconds, and then flows out for five-and-a-half seconds.[3]

When the researchers shifted their attention to the sensors monitoring the blood flow, heart rates, and nervous system activity of their praying subjects, their eyes widened even further. When this slow and steady breath was sustained for a block of time, blood flow to the brain increased. The cardiac and respiratory systems fell into a state of coherence in which the nervous system and all the bodily functions it coordinates worked at peak efficiency. Whenever the subjects interrupted this breathing pattern to talk or attend to other tasks, the integration of these systems slowly fell apart. But it only took a reminder from the researchers, and a few steady breaths for the participants to return to this resonant state.[4]

Ujjayi breathing practiced in this slow and even manner is the best pranayama in which to ground your practice. Traditionally, it's

[3] There is a curious symmetry to these numbers. Breathing in and out for five-and-a-half second intervals results in five-and-a-half breaths per minute, which moves about five-and-a-half liters of air in and out of the lungs.

[4] The traditional yogic way to maintain an even pace of 5-6 breaths per minute was through combining ujjayi pranayama with the mental repetition of a medium-length mantra like Om Ram Shri Ram. Slowly counting out the length of your inbreaths and outbreaths, starting with 1,2,3 and progressing toward 1,2,3,4,5 also works but can become boring. Today there are a number of apps that help users breathe in this rhythm through the use of timers, visual guides, and soothing soundtracks.

the pranayama sustained during yoga poses to synchronize breath and movement, transforming a sequence of bodily postures into an experience of meditation-in-motion. When ujjayi is practiced prior to sitting meditation, it's done differently. The exhalations are gradually extended to twice the length of the inhalations. This uneven breath pattern produces a state of introversion that grants access to a range of meditative states. How these two forms of ujjayi pranayama—the even breath and the doubly long exhalation breath—shift the activity of the autonomic nervous system to produce their disparate results is addressed in Appendix 2.

DIRGHA PRANAYAMA

The word *dirgha* means "long, slow, smooth—all at the same time." The instructions to practice dirgha pranayama can be simply stated. Exhale fully, gently contracting the abdominal muscles as the exhale completes to empty the lungs of residual air. Then take a long, slow, and smooth ujjayi inhalation through the nose, filling the lungs from bottom to top. Once the lungs are filled, shift directly into a long, slow, and smooth ujjayi exhalation, emptying the lungs from top to bottom. As the exhalation is completing, gently squeeze out residual air to set the stage for the next long, slow, and smooth ujjayi inhalation.

Today, dirgha pranayama is often called "three-part breathing" because it teaches you to use the diaphragm to extend the belly forward as the lower lungs are being filled. Then the abdominal muscles engage, which expands the rib cage out to the sides as the mid-lungs are being filled. Finally, the collar bones lift, opening the upper chest and enabling the top of the lungs to be filled. Dirgha pranayama is yoga's way to preserve and expand what doctors call your "vital capacity"—the maximum volume of air a person can exhale after taking the deepest possible inbreath.

The yogis say that only a person able to breathe deeply gets an adequate supply of blood to the head. Today we may express the same idea a little differently. Dirgha pranayama increases blood circulation to all areas of the brain. Its many benefits come from there.

Vital capacity is considered a key measure of respiratory health. In the 1980s, the seventy-year Framingham Study examined 5,200 subjects and found the best indicator of life span was not genetics, diet, or daily exercise, but lung capacity. The University of Buffalo confirmed these results in 2000 by assessing more than a thousand subjects over three decades. Neither of these landmark studies addressed the critical issue for anyone whose capacity has deteriorated: How can I regain full function? That's where dirgha pranayama comes in. The progressive strengthening it provides is yoga's version of weight lifting for the breathing muscles and lungs.

It's easy to take your ability to breathe deeply for granted, but any geriatric doctor will caution you to think differently. People lose a little muscle mass every year starting around age thirty. At the same time, the bones in the chest become thinner, which often causes the rib cage to collapse inward. Both of these age-related changes, especially when coupled with a deficit of vigorous aerobic exercise and targeted torso stretching, can prevent air from easily entering and exiting the body. On top of these biomechanical limitations, the lungs tend to lose about 12% of their gas-exchange capacity from age thirty to fifty. The pace of this decline, if left unchecked, accelerates as we get older, with women faring worse than men due to their smaller chest cavity. The end result is that an average eighty-year-old is able to take in 30% less air than a comparable person in their twenties. This compels them to breathe faster and harder, a respiratory pattern known to lead to serious health problems including hypertension, autoimmune conditions, metabolic issues often associated with weight gain and type two diabetes, and mood disorders. Fortunately, science is proving what yoga has known for millennia. Aging doesn't have to be a steep path of physical decline.

Until the 1980s, doctors believed the reduction in efficiency of internal organs like the lungs was an immutable fact of nature. It's now known that even the condition of the lungs is malleable, as demonstrated by adults who have taught themselves to breathe in ways that increased their vital capacity an astounding 30 to 40%. And the benefit better breathing brings is not confined to bodily health. Research has shown that breathing practices can improve emotional control, enhancing our ability for "self-regulation," and reducing the symptoms of mental conditions including anxiety, depression, insomnia, PTSD, and attention deficit disorder.

OVERBREATHING

Practicing pranayama can leave you feeling zippy or even euphoric, and it's easy for those good feelings to translate into a naive mindset with known downsides. The line of thought that leads into this pitfall goes something like this. "Before, I wasn't breathing enough. Now, I'm breathing more and feeling better. If I can just remember to breathe deep and full all the time, I would have lots of energy and feel great!" Unfortunately, walking the yogic path toward better breathing requires a more sophisticated understanding of pranayama's role. Chronically feeding the body more air than it needs is detrimental to the health of the whole system. The common name for this malady is overbreathing.

Pranayama is not a discipline to help you mentally manipulate the 22,000 breaths you take each day. Attempting that is a surefire recipe for overbreathing and stress! Pranayama is something you do for short periods of time, ideally as an integral part of your daily yoga practice. It's a type of *training* that bestows immediate benefits, but whose greatest value lies in its ability to shift the default mode of your breathing pattern in a healthier direction. Without a doubt, it can be helpful to do short stints of various breathing exercises throughout the day to relax and reset the system, but the goal of pranayama practice is not to practice any formulaic breath pattern round the clock. It's to regain the ability to breathe in a relaxed and free-flowing manner that is responsive to changing circumstances and calibrated by nature to efficiently meet and not exceed your actual metabolic needs.

You can think of the yogic pranayamas as a set of tools a mechanic might use to maintain the engine of a sportscar. The basic ujjayi breath is a way to keep your metabolic engine in good timing. Dirgha breathing keeps it firing powerfully on all cylinders, which is important because every high-performing sportscar needs the ability to accelerate quickly and cruise along easily at highway speeds. A really topnotch engine idles at a very low rate of revolutions per minute. That fine tuning occurs as an increasingly soft ujjayi breath with lengthening exhalations carries you into meditation. Using this analogy, overbreathing is a bit like driving around town revving your engine and wasting fuel. Biochemically, overbreathing offloads too much carbon dioxide from the lungs, which reduces the amount of this chemical below the healthy levels needed to transport oxygen from the bloodstream into the cells.

BE A DISCERNING STUDENT

Scientists the world over are discovering that breathing does much more than supply our cells with oxygen and eliminate excess carbon dioxide and other gaseous wastes. The way we breathe informs our internal organs, telling them when to turn on and off, dramatically affecting our bodily health. It sets our heart rate, influences our hormone levels, and helps determine the speed of our brain waves, which impacts our state of mind. It does all these and many other things in orchestration with the autonomic nervous system or ANS, a network of nerves permeating the body that control all of our involuntary processes.

The ANS got its name based upon a presumption that all its processes were automatic, a proverbial black box entirely outside of our conscious control. But this twentieth-century paradigm is quickly being replaced by a more empowering idea that tracks with the teachings of yoga. Respiration's dual nature as a voluntary and involuntary process enables a person to steer the ANS by regulating the breath in ways that support health, hike resilience, and shift consciousness. The implications of this paradigm shift on yoga practice are enormous. Our discussion of pranayama and the ANS continues in Appendix 2.

APPLYING THIS IN PRACTICE

Swami Kripalu's daily prescription to uplevel vital capacity and boost mood makes scientific sense. Begin with a few minutes of relaxed and rhythmic ujjayi pranayama to warm up your breathing muscles. Gradually shift into a period of dirgha breathing, emptying the lungs from top to bottom, then filling them from bottom to top. After a dozen or more of these full, flowing breaths, close your pranayama session with several minutes of focused ujjayi breathing. You can equalize the length of inbreaths and outbreaths to a slow count of four or five to optimize the workings of all your bodily systems and center yourself, or gradually lengthen out your exhalations to spend a few minutes in spacious meditation. Either way, this whole process can be done in fifteen minutes to great effect.

Pranayamas that slow the breath draw the senses inward. Practicing them, you discover that all forms of mental turmoil are happening outside the cave of your innermost mind. Inside that cave it is always peaceful, which is why these pranayamas are used to enter meditation. Meditation will lead you to the true realization that this innermost mind of yours merges into the soul, but don't get ahead of yourself. The first step is learning how to do these pranayamas, and then practicing them systematically until your good health and peace of mind has been restored.

APPENDIX 2

PRANAYAMA AND THE AUTONOMIC NERVOUS SYSTEM

New life permeates every cell as pranayama is practiced intelligently and the nervous system returns to its natural function.

Anyone intent on practicing pranayama today should study the reciprocal relationship between breathing and the autonomic nervous system or "ANS." This need to couple practice with a conceptual map showing how different breathing patterns affect the body and mind is nothing new. Aspirants of old gained this understanding through yoga's traditional model of the subtle body. Swami Kripalu delves into the intricacies of this model in his commentary on the Hatha Yoga Pradipika, but for most practical purposes it is anachronistic. Today's yogis are likely to find medical science a better starting place. That's especially true when neuroscientists are publishing papers that see pranayama as more than a method of breath control and instead describe it as a sophisticated system of autonomic training the restores the natural self-regulating rhythms of the heart, breath, and mind.

The ANS is a network of nerves originating in the spinal cord and permeating the body that governs our involuntary processes.[1] It's easy to imagine these nerves as the electrical connections the brain requires to coordinate the function of the organs and hormone-secreting glands. But the ANS is a lot more complex than wiring and firing. It has relays that trigger reflexes, and also uses chemical compounds to send important signals, with the neurons switching back and forth between electrical and chemical communication as needed. The ANS extends to the

[1] Autonomic means "self-governing" and describes the somewhat mysterious mechanism regulating all the bodily processes operating outside of our conscious control.

eyes; the throat and voice box; the skin; the heart and vascular system; lungs; the stomach, intestines, colon and rectum; the liver, pancreas, and spleen; the kidneys and adrenals; the bladder and urinary tract; the immune and lymphatic systems; and the sex organs. This synopsis of its extensive reach shows why the ANS is so critical to everyone's health and well-being.

The ANS includes two branches that operate in a see-saw fashion. Its sympathetic branch or "Activating Side" sends signals that excite our system and ready us to take action. When mildly or moderately aroused, it's responsible for the good energy that focuses attention, heightens awareness, sharpens sense perceptions, reduces reaction time, and otherwise enables us to perform well physically and mentally. If strongly triggered, it is the source of the fight or flight response that initiates a cascade of physiological processes to help us escape an imminent physical threat or avoid intense mental distress. To produce this response, the neurotransmitter noradrenaline and a mix of what are often called "stress chemicals" enter the bloodstream to boost the heart rate, increase blood pressure, open the airways of the lungs, and direct blood flow to the skeletal muscles. These chemical messengers also suppress digestion and peristalsis, along with a range of other critical but non-acute health maintenance activities. While triggered at a moment's notice, it takes an hour or more to ramp down from a strong sympathetic activation and fully turn off the flight or fight response.

The parasympathetic branch has the opposite effect. This "Relaxing Side" of the ANS sends signals that soothe the system and help it return to a state of homeostasis after activity. When strongly engaged, this branch is the source of the rest and digest response that enables the body to recover from a stressful encounter and resume healthy functioning.[2] To produce this response, the neurotransmitter acetylcholine and a mix of what are often called "feel-good chemicals" enter the bloodstream to open up attention, decrease the heart rate, lower blood pressure, direct blood flow to digestion and the other vital organs, prompt salivation, ease urination, loosen the bowels, and perform essential bodily functions

[2] The existence of a "relaxation response" was proven by Herbert Benson, MD in the 1970s. "Rest and digest" is a more current term for the same state, and its often used interchangeably with yet another shorthand moniker, the "feed and breed" response, thus named because parasympathetic dominance whets the appetite and facilitates sexual arousal.

during periods of safety and calm. Many reparative functions critical to health only occur in the sound sleep that happens when a person is in a robust state of parasympathetic dominance. Where fight or flight can be triggered quickly, the rest and digest response comes on slowly. It can be facilitated by an assortment of relaxation techniques but generally takes twenty minutes or more to fully engage.

While often described as being in opposition, it's more accurate to see these two sides of the ANS as working together to maintain an optimal internal environment. When one is dominant, the other is more or less suppressed, with the body shifting between degrees of these two states to adapt to changing situations. Humans evolved to spend the majority of their waking hours and all of their sleeping hours in a relaxed state of parasympathetic dominance. Our bodies are built to stay in a state of high sympathetic arousal for shorts bursts, and only on occasion. Otherwise, we're subject to all the difficulties associated with prolonged stress and the malady commonly known as "burn out."

The Activating Side of the ANS has gotten a bad rap in the press, even though its proper functioning is just as vital to our well-being as its Relaxing Side partner. That's because in our postmodern world of paper tigers, it is relatively rare to encounter a life-threatening situation requiring a full-blown fight or flight response, and all too common to suffer from stress and burnout. As the author James Nestor writes, many of us "spend our days half-asleep and our nights half-awake, lolling in a grey zone of half-anxiety. During these times, the organs throughout the body won't be shut down, but will instead be supported in a state of suspended animation; blood flow will decrease and communication between the organs and the brain will become choppy, like a conversation through a staticky phone line. Our bodies can persist like this for a while; they can keep us alive, but they can't keep us healthy."[3]

Dysautonomia is the medical name for this condition, which technically isn't a disease but a catch-all category for an array of symptoms that result when both sides of the ANS are unable to play their roles effectively. This includes dizziness, fainting, problems with heart rate and blood pressure, chronic fatigue, digestive difficulties, metabolic syndrome,[4] trouble regulating body temperature, and a range of

[3] *Breath: The New Science of a Lost Art* (Riverhead Books, 2020), 149.

[4] Research links ANS dysfunction to metabolic syndrome, an increasingly prevalent

autoimmune disorders. Over 70 million people worldwide are believed to suffer from some form of dysautonomia. Because it can take so many forms, dysautonomia is a difficult condition for healthcare providers to diagnose, which means it often goes untreated.

ANS GEAR SHIFTING

Understanding the autonomic nervous system can shed a lot of light on the practice of pranayama, but only after a common misperception has been corrected. As its name signifies, the ANS has always been thought to operate automatically and outside of our conscious control. None of us can *directly* alter our blood chemistry, control our heartbeat, and turn our organ systems on or off. But researchers are discovering that virtually all of us can do these things *indirectly* through techniques that signal the ANS to shift gears. By far the quickest, the most effective, and the easiest of these techniques to learn is consciously regulating the breath.

Let's explore how this can work with the foundational pranayamas beginning with ujjayi breathing. The lungs are covered with a profusion of nerve fibers connected to the ANS. Most of the nerves tracing back to the Activating Side are spread across the top of the lungs. These nerves are sensitive to both the pace and volume of the inbreath. Taking in the kind of strong and full inhalation you might begin a cardiovascular workout with stimulates these nerves, which excites the system, increases the heart rate, warms the body, and speeds up metabolism to provide you with needed energy. Unfortunately, those same nerves are constantly being stimulated whenever you take the short, shallow, and hasty breaths characteristic of upper chest breathing. Unknowingly, you are signaling your body to uplevel its Activating Side activity. Over time a breath pattern like this overtaxes the ANS and is likely to produce the aforementioned "grey zone of half-anxiety" associated with dysautonomia.

Most of the nerves connected to the Relaxing Side are located in the lower lungs. When air flows easily into the lungs via a diaphragmatic

---

cluster of conditions including high blood pressure, high blood sugar, excess belly fat, and abnormal cholesterol/triglyceride levels that increase the risk of heart disease, stroke, and type 2 diabetes. Studies have shown that people with metabolic syndrome often exhibit overly high sympathetic activity, but more research is needed to understand the link between metabolic syndrome and dysautonomia. Dysautonomia is often linked to low functioning of the vagus nerve—see page 272.

inbreath, these nerves signal your body that it's safe to rest and digest. But this is only half the reason belly breathing feels so relaxing. As the air exits the lower lungs on the outbreath, it stimulates a second parasympathetic response. This doubling mechanism explains the tranquilizing effects of all the pranayamas that lengthen the outbreath. The upshot of these nerve responses is simple but far reaching. The softer and slower you breathe in using the muscles of the diaphragm so as to not excite the Activating Side, and the longer you exhale by relaxing the belly to doubly engage the Relaxing Side, the more slowly the heart beats, the calmer you feel, and the better your organ function and thus overall health.

A pragmatic understanding of the above anatomy is built into ujjayi pranayama. Practice begins by gently constricting the throat to make the ujjayi sound, which simultaneously softens the inbreath and extends the outbreath. If you are feeling stressed, this will help you step back and not go over the cliff of fight-or-flight triggering. Ujjayi pranayama continues its work as you equalize the length of your inbreaths and outbreaths, which establishes the balanced state of ANS functioning that bestows a relaxed and attentive focus. A yoga practitioner using ujjayi breathing to enter deep relaxation or meditation will gradually extend the exhalation until it is about twice as long as the inhalation. Along with all the health benefits of engaging the rest and digest response, this breathing pattern further slows the heart rate and introverts the mind. As outer distractions fall away, relaxation and meditation come easily.

DIRGHA PRANAYAMA

While the primary bodily benefit of practicing dirgha pranayama is stretching and strengthening your breathing muscles to preserve your rib cage flexibility and vital capacity, it also affects the ANS in a distinctive way that plays an important role in yoga practice.

Dirgha pranayama begins with a long ujjayi exhalation in which the lungs are emptied by a full relaxation of the dome-shaped diaphragm, after which the residual air is squeezed out of the lungs through a gentle contraction of the abdominal muscles. This powerfully stimulates the nerves in the lower lungs associated with the Relaxing Side of the ANS. The long and slow ujjayi inhalation that follows extends all the way to the collar bones, which mildly stimulates the nerves in the upper chest associated with the Activating Side of the ANS. But that stimulation is modest in degree, and it's immediately followed by another long, slow, and full exhalation that doubly stimulates the Relaxing Side.

By activating both sides of the ANS in a way that ensures parasympathetic dominance, dirgha pranayama produces a state of energized calm. The boost in energy that results from ten to fifteen minutes of its practice feels a little like drinking a good cup of coffee and is a great preparation for the practice of yoga postures. It can also be used to energize the body before returning to ujjayi breathing or shifting to nadi shodhana, both of which soften the inhalations and lengthen the exhalations to ready the mind for meditation.

NADI SHODHANA

A little more ANS knowledge is required to explain the effects of alternate nostril breathing. Let's start with its simplest expression called nadi shodhana, which for these purposes can be thought of as ujjayi pranayama through alternating nostrils.

Medicine has long known the breath naturally oscillates from nostril to nostril in a pattern known as the nasal cycle. Approximately every two hours, what is called the dominant nostril switches back and forth. At any given moment, about seventy-five percent of our breathing is taking place through one nostril and twenty-five percent from the other. Doctors are still debating why the nasal cycle occurs. Yogis say this natural oscillation is an important way the body maintains a healthy state of balance, and current ANS research suggests that is correct.

Breathing through the right nostril activates the sympathetic or Activating Side of the ANS that signals the body-mind to enter an elevated state of alertness and action-readiness. The author James Nestor likens this to pressing down the gas pedal of your car. In response, cortisol levels rise slightly and your heart rate, temperature, and blood pressure increase. Right nostril breathing also feeds blood to the left hemisphere of the brain and its pre-frontal cortex, which narrows the beam of your attention to improve analytical thinking and support decisive action.

Breathing through the left nostril activates the parasympathetic or Relaxing Side of the ANS that signals the body-mind to return to a relaxed state of homeostasis. In response, acetylcholine levels rise slightly, the body cools, and your heart rate and blood pressure decrease. This is the equivalent of pressing on the brake, which shifts blood flow to the right hemisphere of the brain. This broadens the beam of your attention to enhance creativity and support the holistic thinking that views everything as an interconnected whole.

Our bodies and minds operate at peak efficiency in the precious few moments of nervous system balance that naturally occur at the midpoint of the nasal cycle. That's where the practice of nadi shodhana comes in. It provides a simple way to intentionally bring yourself into that balanced state. The yogic texts call the flow of breath through the right nostril the *solar pathway*, and the flow of breath through the left nostril the *lunar pathway*. Breathing through alternate nostrils is said to equalize the flow of energy in these two pathways. Poised in mental equilibrium, with both sides of the ANS and brain moderately engaged, a yoga practitioner finds it easier to simultaneously focus attention and relax into meditation.

The energy channel controlled by the right nostril is called the fiery flow. The energy channel controlled by the left nostril is called the cooling flow. Sometimes the breath flows more forcefully through the right side. Other times it flows more forcefully through the left side. When it flows with equal force through both nostrils, it is called "the very kind flow" because in this state the whole being finds balance and contemplation comes easily. Understanding the subtlety of this relationship between the right and left nostrils is an esoteric secret of yoga.

KAPALABHATI

Kapalabhati breathing has been the subject of multiple scientific studies. Together the research findings show that its practice enhances general health and fitness along with providing an impressive list of discrete benefits. Kapalabhati improves lung function, increases overall respiratory efficiency, shifts cerebral blood flow in ways that enhance attention and focus, reduces anxiety, positively impacts heart rate variability, and raises the body's basal metabolic rate in a way that reduces fat deposits and aids in weight loss. The strength of these preliminary results has led researchers to postulate that kapalabhati breathing may be an intervention capable of combating metabolic syndrome by improving "ANS modulation," which means the ease with which the ANS can smoothly shift its functioning from one side to the other. All these studies acknowledge that additional research is needed to better understand the mechanisms producing these benefits and assess the long-term effects of kapalabhati practice.[5]

Even at this early stage, the researchers have sketched a diagram of how kapalabhati breathing produces a dynamic pattern of ANS activity supportive of health. As little as one minute of practice initiates a cascade of measurable bodily responses that lead to an increase in heart rate, an uptick in systolic and diastolic blood pressure, with various changes in blood chemistry and cerebral blood flow, all of which indicate "an acute phase of sympathetic activation and parasympathetic withdrawal." This quick stimulation of the Activating Side is what generates a practitioner's sense of rising energy, increased alertness, and sharpening mental focus. Once the active phase of kapalabhati breathing completes, a gradual fall off of all these parameters begins that leads to what researchers call a "parasympathetic rebound." After a twenty-minute rest period, a significant state of Relaxing Side dominance was present in all subjects. Researchers posit that this rapid gear shifting from sympathetic to parasympathetic dominance may be the mechanism through which kapalabhati improves ANS modulation and produces many of its health benefits.[6]

[5] Yogis, including SK, describe kapalabhati as purifying the blood. Researchers note a rapid off-loading of carbon dioxide from deoxygenated venous blood which later enhances blood oxygen saturation. Yoga teachers often say that kapalabhati increases blood flow to the brain. The studies show that kapalabhati does alter brain activity, but it accomplishes this by decreasing (versus increasing) cerebral blood flow.

[6] The trending practice of "cold plunges" triggers an interplay of ANS responses similar to kapalabhati. Cold exposure initially stimulates the Activating Side of the ANS, but that is soon followed by an equally strong Relaxing Side response. Repeated cold exposure, like regular kapalabhati practice, forces the ANS to adapt and become more efficient at shifting between states of sympathetic and parasympathetic dominance, improving its ability to regulate the system in the face of stress. Cold plunging can lead to a sudden loss of consciousness or paralysis that poses a real risk of drowning when done in or near bodies of water. Cold showers can have the same or similar effects, and some traditional yoga schools guide students to take one daily, arguably to receive these positive ANS effects.

It's important to highlight several safeguards built into the kapalabhati technique that check its impact on the sympathetic or Activating Side. Together these safeguards prevent it from triggering a full-blown flight-or-fight response. First among them is the instruction to keep the inbreaths relaxed and passive, which avoids over-stimulating the nerves in the upper lungs that excite the Activating Side. Next are the rhythmic contractions of the diaphragm and repetitive strong exhalations, both of which stimulate the nerves in the lower lungs that trace back to the Relaxing Side. When the practice of kapalabhati breathing is done properly and at a restrained pace, it produces a moderate and desirable spike in Activating Side symptoms that quickly trails off into Relaxing Side dominance.

Some seekers encounter deep tensions and do not know how to make their body and mind relaxed. As a result, they feel frustrated and do not succeed in accessing meditative introversion. One aspect of the art of relaxation is counterintuitive. Undergoing laborious activities, the bodily organs and nerves grow fatigued. When the labors end, they automatically slip toward the state of relaxation. This is how an active process like kapalabhati with its quick and successive breaths can be used to generate a shift into deep relaxation. A seeker who understands this natural interplay of effort and relaxation has obtained an important key for attaining introversion.

BE A DISCERNING STUDENT

In response to the growing interest in breathwork, a new professional field is taking shape that calls itself "respiration physiology." In coming decades, it's likely a steady stream of research papers will be published that have direct implications for pranayama practice. But science as a rule moves slowly, and the researchers currently working in the field describe themselves as only scratching the surface. Until greater clarity emerges, yoga practitioners will be forced to rely on pragmatic models like those presented in this appendix, which endeavor to utilize the scientific information available but remain decidedly heuristic in nature.

APPLYING THIS IN PRACTICE

Cutting-edge science agrees with age-old yogic wisdom in concluding that breathing exercises which slow, smooth, and lengthen the breath are generally safe and beneficial. The same cannot be said of pranayamas that forcefully pump the breath or involve extended breath holding. These require proper and progressive training to master and have known contraindications, especially for those who have experienced trauma or otherwise are prone to anxiety or panic attacks. A discerning student remains aware that the benefits and possible detriments of these practices are not yet fully understood. Knowing this, they seek expert guidance and carefully monitor the results of their practice. In questionable areas, they choose to exercise caution.

People often ask me how yogic pranayama works, which I will now explain to you in brief. The yogis of old observed that underneath our most powerful feelings is a bodily energy that throws the mind in a single direction. We all have gotten angry at someone and become so engrossed in our story of being wronged that all other thoughts are forgotten. The same can be said of sexual arousal, terror, and grief. The yogis of old learned through regulating the flow of breath that the same energy underlying these powerful feelings can be directed to higher levels where it becomes equally beautiful. That's the purpose of pranayama—to bring forth this bodily generated one-pointed focus without creating any disturbance in the mind.

APPENDIX 3

UNDERSTANDING THE ADVANCED PRANAYAMAS

It is said that a healthy yogic aspirant should practice ujjayi and dirgha pranayama along with moderate diet for some months before beginning nadi shodhana. Nadi shodhana should be practiced for many months before starting kapalabhati and anuloma viloma. One should do these pranayamas moderately and not be too enthusiastic in increasing either the time or depth of practice. In the yoga system of the ancient sages, pranayama practice beyond this point was only initiated through the guidance of a discerning guru.

As just explained, a powerful mechanism called the autonomic nervous system underlies much of pranayama's effectiveness. One health-related goal of breathing practice is learning how to use pranayama to turn off the fight-or-flight response and turn on the rest-and-digest response by bringing the ANS into a state of parasympathetic dominance. A second is to improve ANS modulation by improving its ability to smoothly shift back and forth between its Activating and Relaxing Sides to improve stress resilience. A third goal is using pranayama to bring the ANS into a balanced state that sharpens the mental focus so useful in modern life and is equally supportive of meditation and spiritual growth.

All three of these goals carry forward into the practice of the advanced pranayamas, but the mechanisms through which they are pursued changes. Understanding the biology underlying these techniques, even if they are never applied in practice, will expand your knowledge of how all of the classical yogic pranayamas work.

Many diseases of the body are destroyed by the foundational pranayamas. But some diseases hide themselves deep in our fears. It is for these conditions that the advanced pranayamas are taught to aspirants possessing the strong constitution required to practice them.

ANULOMA VILOMA

Anuloma viloma is not a single practice. There are three major variations, the first two of which were presented in Chapter Ten. The third was presented in Chapter 12 under the name Swami Kripalu used to distinguish it: *sahita kumbhak*. The first of these anuloma viloma variations can be thought of as "dirgha pranayama through alternating nostrils." These are slow and smooth inbreaths and outbreaths that fill and empty the lungs. At the end of every inhalation is a relaxing pause in which the flow of breath naturally ceases. It's during this pendulum-like pause that the breath is manually shifted to the opposite nostril. The effect of this momentary stoppage of the breath, which is actually a brief breath hold, should not be ignored. After holding the breath for even a second, the subsequent exhalation is accompanied by a noticeably heightened feeling of tension release.

We have already seen how a three-part dirgha inbreath taken all the way to the upper chest mildly stimulates the Activating Side of the ANS and is thus experienced as energy arousing. It's the same for these dirgha-like breaths, which are now being taken through alternating nostrils. Breathing in and out through a single nostril further slows the pace of each breath, which increases the double Relaxing Side stimulation that occurs on each exhalation. It also brings into play the brain balancing effects of nadi shodhana. For all these reasons, anuloma viloma practiced as dirgha pranayama through alternating nostrils produces a paradoxical state of heightened energy, strong mental focus, and bodily relaxation.

The next variation of anuloma viloma introduces the practice of systematic breath holding. This adds a strong ANS-modulating dynamic to the technique. The first step is to synchronize the phases of the breath—inhalation, hold, exhalation—as to their duration. This is no longer "dirgha pranayama through alternating nostrils" because the length of the inbreath is markedly shorter. The inhale flows in naturally and unforced, which probably means to a count of three or four, perhaps a little longer for regular practitioners. The breath is then "held to capacity," which is defined as "exhaling when reaching your comfort level." The exhale flows out smoothly, free of any discomfort or gasping for air that can come if the breath is held too long, to a count approximately twice as long as the inhalation. As the different phases of the breath come into synch, it's possible to relax deeply into what feels like a meditative practice.

Once a practitioner's body acquaints itself to this process, the initial moments of breath holding are experienced as calming. The nervous system quiets and the mind slows. As carbon dioxide levels start to rise, the body tries to compensate for the lack of oxygen it anticipates may be coming by activating what is called the *baroreflex*. This reflex rapidly decreases the heart rate and blood pressure to maintain a stable amount of oxygen delivery to the system. As breath-holding continues, two things can occur. Practitioners in training will reach the limit of their comfort level. They have "held to capacity" and it's time for them to exhale. Experienced practitioners doing the technique in a relaxed and meditative manner are likely to trigger the *mammalian dive reflex* that further slows the heart rate, directs blood to essential organs, and allows for extended holding. Activating either or both of these reflexes powerfully stimulates the Relaxing Side of the ANS.[1]

Sage Patanjali delineates the phases of respiration. The first is the outflow of breath (rechaka), the second is the inflow of breath

[1] The baroreflex is an internal mechanism that acts quickly to regulate blood pressure (BP). When baroreceptors located in the blood vessel walls sense an increase in BP due to breath holding, they signal the brain to decrease the heart rate and dilate blood vessels, both of which lower BP. The mammalian dive reflex (MDR) is an unconscious physiological reaction triggered by submersion in water that can also be activated by intentional breath-holding. It further slows the heart rate and directs blood flow to essential organs by constricting peripheral blood vessels. While the MDR has some therapeutic applications, it also has risks especially for those with underlying heart conditions, and its overall impact upon health is not yet understood. Some sources I found link it with the mysterious phenomenon known as "sudden death syndrome." Serious and in this instance potentially fatal contraindications require careful consideration, especially when they are reflected in the traditional warnings issued to practitioners against the overzealous, uninformed, and unsupervised practice of advanced pranayama and especially breath-holding techniques.

(puraka), and the third is the checked breath (kumbhaka). A yogi in the middle stage of pranayama gives equal importance to exhaling, inhaling, and holding. A yogi advancing in pranayama toward the states of dharana and dhyana makes a deliberate effort to extend their ability to hold the breath to bring stability to the mental faculty.

All practitioners will eventually sense their comfort level approaching and reach what is called their "breath holding breakpoint." In these final moments of holding, the need to breathe is registered as a stressor.[2] This powerfully stimulates the Activating Side of the ANS, which signals the body to increase the heart rate and blood pressure. But that nascent activation is quickly quelled by the smooth release of the holding via a long and slow exhalation. This ratcheting back and forth between the activating and relaxing sides is the primary mechanism through which this anuloma viloma variation exerts a modulating effect on the ANS.

In a mature practice of anuloma viloma, these two variations come together into a single practice. What starts out as a relatively short inhalation taken to a count of three or four gradually grows longer until it becomes a complete dirgha-like inhalation. As the body becomes accustomed to this practice, that long inbreath can be held progressively longer, until a natural limit of approximately four times the length of the inhalation is reached. A longer inbreath allows for a longer and slower exhalation of roughly twice the inhalation's length. The process of merging these two practices into a mature expression of anuloma viloma is an intensive breath training that must be done slowly. Even in optimal conditions, it takes considerable time for the body's limits to be expanded. Thinking back to my failed attempt at

[2] The feeling of panic that accompanies prolonged breath holding is activated by a cluster of neurons at the base of the brain stem called the chemoreceptors. Flexible chemoreception is part of what distinguishes great athletes, who have trained their chemoreceptors to withstand the extreme fluctuations in carbon dioxide levels that accompany vigorous competition without panicking. Studies show that individuals with certain anxiety-related conditions or trauma have notably low carbon dioxide levels and display a much greater fear of holding their breath. This supports SK's caution and repeated assertions that these breath holding practices can trigger strong emotional reactions and are not for everyone. With almost one in five Americans suffering from anxiety and panic attacks, doctors are exploring whether breath holding protocols similar to those taught in yoga may be able to treat these disorders by conditioning their chemoreceptors to be more flexible.

renunciate pranayama, it's clear I was forcing the process. The aggressive manner in which I was performing anuloma viloma was overstimulating my Activating Side, which kept me in a state of low-grade flight or fight arousal. This had a range of deleterious effects and ultimately forced me to abandon the practice.

Inhale slowly through either one or both nostrils and then retain the breath for as long as comfortable. When a strong urge to exhale arises, slowly and smoothly empty the lungs. This form of pranayama can be practiced for up to fifteen minutes with little fatigue. It is of equal importance to those wanting to regain their health and yogis wanting to realize God. When one smoothly fills the chest and retains the breath, the heart beats slower and slower. This soothes all the vital organs. As the urge to exhale peaks, it sharpens the focus of the mind. The relaxed body and alert mind that results is easily led into meditation. But other effects may occur, as this pranayama causes some individuals to grow lightheaded, faint, fall into trance, or feel mental anguish. This is why pranayamas of this caliber (ones that retain the breath) should only be practiced under the auspices of an experienced guru.

SAHITA KUMBHAK

In the most advanced variation of anuloma viloma, which SK distinguished as *sahita kumbhak*, the inbreath is held until the practitioner feels "compelled to release the breath." Although the effect of this change is relatively minor in terms of time duration, it extends the holding beyond the practitioner's comfort level, which dramatically amplifies the degree of ANS volatility generated by the practice. A second shorter but equally ardent holding out of the breath at the end of the exhalation may also be added, which further intensifies the practice. I am not aware of any scientific studies on point, but here is my practitioner's perspective on how this intensive technique works informed by the principles that research has identified.[3]

[3] At present, there is no scientific explanation of the breath-holding breakpoint that integrates all the various factors known to play a role. Although the breath can be

The initial phases of sahita kumbhak affect the ANS in the same way as mature practice of anuloma viloma. As the breath is held in, the system calms and both the baroreflex and mammalian dive reflex respond to slow the heart rate. This is where the techniques part ways. As the breath continues to be held beyond the practitioner's comfort level, a sense of urgency arises that can be suppressed for a time but eventually moves in the direction of panic. This strong reaction reveals that the Activating Side of the ANS has engaged and its flight or fight response is on the verge of being triggered. When the held breath is finally released in a long and slow exhalation, the panic abates and the system calms, but the relief is short-lived. In the next hold the panic returns, until it is again quelled by a long and slow outbreath, after which yet another hold is engaged. An attentive reader might imagine this rapid fire switching back and forth between extreme degrees of Activating Side and Relaxing Side engagement might be done to improve ANS modulation, but I personally don't think this practice as traditionally practiced has anything to do with promoting bodily health.

An ardent spiritual practitioner making a determined effort to acclimate to this intensive practice by necessity undergoes a rigorous mental training in which high levels of bodily distress and nervous system disturbance must be tolerated. SK said the purpose of this training was "stabilizing the mental faculty." But he also cited the yogic texts that describe this practice as opening a portal into swoons, trances, and non-ordinary mind states.[4] You may recall my story of performing a simple variant of sahita kumbhak while hiking the Appalachian Trail and the dream-like vision it produced. Eventually, the mental strengthening sought in this rigorous breath-holding is gained. When this occurs, the focus of a yogi's practice is meant to shift to samyama and the next three stages of yoga,

held voluntarily, normal individuals are unable to hold the breath to unconsciousness. An involuntary mechanism overrides the willful holding. The occurrence of this breakpoint does not appear to solely be the result of lung mechanisms, the pressure or composition of blood gases, any need for oxygen, or input from the chemoreceptors. Studies suggest a "central respiratory rhythm" generated in the brainstem continues throughout breath-holding. Although this rhythm can be temporarily suppressed, it cannot be stopped voluntarily, and eventually reasserts itself well before oxygen deprivation factors into the equation.

[4] Tirumalai Krishnamacharya (1888-1989) was a contemporary of SK who is credited with founding the modern Ashtangha Yoga lineage. He taught a similar form of advanced pranayama in these verses: "Inhale, and God approaches you. Hold the inhalation, and God remains with you. Exhale, and you approach God. Hold the exhalation, and surrender to God."

in which this strength of mind is helpful in accessing the full range of meditative states that lie beyond pranayama.

An adept yogi commencing the practice of sahita kumbhak suspends the breath again and again until drops of sweat appear. Continuing in this practice, the breath is suspended until a type of shuddering occurs. Through this practice, forbearance develops, and a yogi becomes stable in wisdom. But this pranayama is not for ordinary aspirants. If wrongly undertaken, the inner heat increases, the bodily humors deviate from their natural state, and the whole system is thrown into upset.

BHASTRIKA PRANAYAMA

Bhastrika or bellows breathing differs from all the other pranayamas in a way that sounds crazy. Bhastrika excites the Activating Side of the ANS to a degree that quickly triggers the fight-or-flight response. In order to understand how inducing what medicine calls "sympathetic nervous system overload" could possibly be beneficial, you have to know a bit about the vagus nerve.

The word vagus means "wandering," a description of the meandering path taken by this longest of the cranial nerves as it exits the brain stem and winds through the neck, chest, and abdomen to form a hard-wire link between the brain and all the major organ systems. The vagus nerve is sometimes characterized as an information superhighway. In one direction, it carries vital sensory information from the body to the brain. In the other, it delivers motor commands from the brain to a myriad of organ and gland-related muscles. The critical thing to know for our discussion of yogic pranayama is that the vagus nerve is a key component of the parasympathetic nervous system. It's what turns the organs and glands on and off in response to stress.

The significant impact of the vagus nerve on health has been extensively studied as summarized in the footnote.[5] To help interpret these

[5] Cardiovascular: The vagus helps regulate respiration, heart rate, blood pressure, and body temperature. Good vagal function is associated with a lower resting heart rate, reduced blood pressure, and overall heart/lung health. Digestive health: The

findings, researchers have developed the concept of "vagal tone." A person who displays symptoms associated with a robustly functioning vagus nerve is said to have a high vagal tone. A person who displays symptoms linked to its compromised function is said to have a low vagal tone. Vagal tone is more than a theory. It can be measured indirectly through physiological tests including heart rate variability (HRV) and respiratory sinus arrhythmia (RSA). In general, a high vagal tone reflects a healthy ANS able to weather incidents of stress and quickly return the system to a restorative state of Relaxing Side dominance. A low vagal tone suggests an imbalance in the ANS, most often a chronic state of Activating Side dominance that is impairing organ function.

All of the slow-and-smooth pranayamas discussed earlier soothe the ANS into a state of Relaxing Side dominance that opens the communication lines of the vagal network, which allows the brainstem to better regulate the system. Bhastrika accomplishes the same end goal, but through an exaggerated sequence of steps that make the abstract notion of improving vagal tone easier to grasp. In describing bhastrika like practices, author James Nestor writes, "Simpler and less intense methods of breathing slow, less, and through the nose with a big exhale, can diffuse stress and restore balance. [But] sometimes the body needs more than a soft nudge to get realigned. Sometimes it needs a violent shove" (page 148).

The vigorous series of full inhalations flowing directly into full

---

vagus is a key component of the "gut-brain axis." It regulates the release of digestive enzymes, gastric acid, and bile, and controls the contractions that empty the stomach and move food through the digestive tract. Good vagal function manages blood sugar levels and produces stable energy. Impairments can lead to a range of gastrointestinal problems including bloating, acid reflux or GERD, and irritable bowel syndrome (IBS). Immune System: By regulating the production of anti-inflammatory compounds, the vagus prevents excessive inflammation and supports your body's ability to fight off infections and heal from injuries. Chronic inflammation is an underlying factor in many diseases including autoimmune disorders such as rheumatoid arthritis, metabolic syndrome, and neurodegenerative conditions like Alzheimer's. Swallowing and Speech: These are complex muscular actions to coordinate and poor vagal function can lead to spasms, chronic throat tickles or coughs, and difficulty maintaining or changing vocal pitch. Mental Health: The influence the vagus exerts on the brain, particularly through the gut-brain axis, plays a significant role in mood regulation. Good vagal function is associated with stress hardiness and lower rates of anxiety, depression, poor sleep, brain fog, and headaches including migraines. Cognitive Function: Current research is linking the vagus to cognitive processes including attention, memory, emotional self-regulation, decision-making, and executive function. It is widely accepted that vagal function can be enhanced through practices such as yoga, pranayama, and meditation.

exhalations that constitutes "bellows breathing" flips a switch in the ANS that kicks its Activating Side into high gear. If the breathing is vigorous and sustained, the Relaxing Side, and through it the vagal nerve, is literally shut down.[6] The guiding idea is that doing bhastrika pranayama is like pushing the reset button on your vagus nerve. After being turned off, the vagus nerve will come back online in a way that bestows an opportunity to increase its tone, in much the same way that powering an iPhone on and off restores its factory settings.

There are two ways this reset process can be done in practice. In the simplest version, one or more rounds of bhastrika end with a final inhalation. If you have been doing the common variation in which the arms are raised during inhalation and lowered during exhalations, you inhale the arms overhead. Hold the breath in for ten-to-twenty seconds, and then release it with a long and audible sigh out of the mouth as the arms slowly lower. Once the breath returns to normal, move directly into ujjayi pranayama, gradually lengthening out the exhalations to reengage the Relaxing Side of the ANS and jump start its modulation process.

In the more advanced versions, each round of bhastrika ends with a sustained holding of the breath either in or out, often coupled with various bandhas. Bandhas are subtle muscular contractions, often done in multiple combination, that were traditionally described as directing prana into the major energy channels of the subtle body to activate the chakras and elevate consciousness. Today the bandhas are often explained as techniques to alter the function of the nervous system. If engaged properly after a round of bhastrika pranayama, the bandhas momentarily paralyze the vagal nerve, and the sudden shift back into vagal nerve activity after the contractions are released amplifies the reset process. It is important to understand that both of these ways to end bhastrika build upon the regenerative power of the stress cycle built into us by nature. After the fight-or-flight response enables a prey animal to escape a life-endangering predation threat, the rest-and-digest response is pre-programmed to reassert itself to help the animal recover.

Traditional yoga praises bhastrika pranayama as a method of quickly

[6] It is known that breath-holds of significant duration, especially when coupled with a firming of the diaphragm muscle, can bring about a momentary paralysis of the phrenic motor nerve that controls the diaphragm for purposes of respiration, which acts to extend the breath-holding breakpoint, and bring about a similar paralysis of the vagus nerve.

entering thought-free meditation. Contemporary teachers often explain this by saying that bellows breathing increases oxygen supply to the brain, which enhances concentration and mental clarity. But researchers have proven the exact opposite is true. Whenever the body takes in more air than it needs, carbon dioxide levels drop precipitously, which narrows blood vessels and decreases circulation to the brain. After a minute or more of bhastrika-like breathing, brain blood flow can decrease by forty percent. If the intensive breathing continues, blood drains from the brain and various centers including those that govern time measurement, sense of self, and memory cease to function properly.

For a long time, I practiced three rounds of intensive bhastrika each morning. After each round, I would rest for a few minutes in the state of inner silence this generated. I still do bhastrika pranayama for its invigorating effects. And I am aware that research has clearly shown that various meditative states are produced by stimulating certain brain areas and networks, and notably diminishing the activity of others. But after learning the mechanics through which bhastrika produces what could be called "a blank mind," I ceased doing it for the purpose of entering meditation.

Pranayama frees the nervous system of inhibiting blocks and allows it to coordinate the work of all the organs, especially the nutrition-providing and waste eliminating digestive system. Numberless are the diseases that can be remedied by this approach. Sluggishness of the body-mind comes from a lethargic nervous system and may be called depression. A frenzied body-mind comes from an overwrought nervous system and may be called anxiety. Pranayama restores responsiveness to the nervous system so peace of mind and the vitality of the individual can be regained. When the mind entrains with a healthy body, our shallowness decreases, and the depth of our humanity comes forth. Indeed, it is only through a multiplication of this individual process that society at large can advance toward greatness.

BHRAMARI PRANAYAMA

It's nice to end our lengthy discussion of the yogic pranayamas with a breathing exercise that brings many of the benefits bestowed by its advanced techniques with none of their cautions or contraindications. Bhramari pranayama is a simple and almost effortless practice. You breathe in a long inhalation through the nose. Keeping the lips sealed, you breathe out a very long exhalation through the nose while making a humming sound. Yoga has long praised bhramari pranayama for its ability to relax the body and tranquilize the mind. Now there's an extensive body of research supporting those claims and suggesting the mechanisms through which its benefits are produced.

Bhramari pranayama or what the researchers call "bumble bee breath" has been shown to improve cardiovascular health by simultaneously lowering heart rate and blood pressure, and upleveling lung function and respiratory efficiency. Several studies demonstrate improvements in cognitive function through better attentional control and sleep quality. Consistent practitioners display enhanced mood, better emotional regulation, and lower levels of stress, anxiety, depression, and insomnia. The complete list of benefits was notable enough to motivate the National Institutes of Health to formally review the scientific literature and post on its website that the evidence provides "a very strong case for making bumble bee breath a daily practice for healthy individuals." Instead of stopping there, the NIH went on to recommend that integrative medical providers explore how this practice, given its simplicity and apparent scope of benefits, could be utilized "as a public health lifestyle intervention for disease prevention and improved quality of life."

How does bhramari pranayama deliver all these benefits? The studies suggest it works through a trio of mechanisms. The first of these is no surprise. Bhramari breathing—presumably by virtue of its extended exhalation—curbs the Activating Side of the ANS and stimulates its Relaxing Side partner. The research shows that regular practitioners succeed in engaging the rest-and-digest response and end their practice in a state of parasympathetic nervous system dominance with all its attendant health benefits. In discussing the role of this mechanism in Bumble Bee Breath's effectiveness, the NIH notes that similar benefits are known to result from other breathing exercises, biofeedback training, and regular yoga practice.

A second mechanism amplifies bhramari pranayama's salutary effect on the ANS. It appears the physical vibrations produced by the humming exhalation stimulate the auricular branch of the vagus nerve, which runs through the throat, chest, and head connecting the ears to the brainstem. The brainstem receives these vagus nerve impulses, which activates the parasympathetic nervous system by triggering the rest-and-digest response. This vibratory effect may be the secret to the efficacy of this easy and non-taxing pranayama. It may also explain two other benefits identified by the research but not yet understood. Bhramari breathing increases the proportion of gamma waves in the brain, which are linked to better cognitive function, learning, and mental focus. It also leads to the release of endorphins to a degree that not only enhances mood but led the NIH to ask if these "natural painkillers" could potentially help post-surgery patients in their recovery.

The third mechanism factoring into bhramari's effectiveness is the tremendous increase in nitric oxide generated by its practice. Nitric oxide is essential to health, and our sinuses and nasal passages are constantly producing it. Nitric oxide is a vasodilator, which means it opens blood vessels to improve circulation and oxygen transport. The humming exhalations through the nose create air oscillations that increase the production of nitric oxide fifteen-fold as compared to a normal exhalation. The additional nitric oxide enters the bloodstream, where it promotes heart health and aids oxygen delivery throughout the body. Nitric oxide is also known to play a role in brain health and function, and increased levels may improve memory along with a range of cognitive abilities. Finally, nitric oxide is an anti-inflammatory that helps the immune system defend against bacterial, viral, fungal, and parasitic infections to a degree that led the NIH to speculate that bumble bee breath might be able to play a role in the treatment of COVID-19.

BE A DISCERNING STUDENT

While researching the effects of yogic breathing, I kept running into studies reporting that the practice of pranayama "improved heart rate variability." The authors were quick to point out that "HRV" was a generally accepted measure of stress hardiness and vagal tone, but failed to explain anything further. That left me wondering. Is heart rate variability a good thing or a bad thing? Definitively answering this question revolutionized my understanding of yogic pranayama.

HRV measures the subtle fluctuations in the time interval between adjacent heartbeats. Learning this led me to immediately assume that good health would show up as a steady resting heart rate, but I quickly found out otherwise. Small variations in the time interval between heartbeats show that the body is poised to adapt to changing situations. Underlying that poise is a nimble ANS able to smoothly shift back and forth between its activating and relaxing sides to raise and lower heart rate and hormone levels as needed. This explains why doctors consider HRV a proxy for vagal tone. When a person's vagus nerve is strongly functioning, their heart rate varies from beat to beat in this fashion.[7]

Understanding HRV took my inquiry deeper. If true well-being is not a steady homeostatic state, but more a matter of agile responsiveness, what is the role of pranayama in fostering health? My mind circled back to the SK quote opening Appendix 2: *New life permeates every cell as pranayama is practiced intelligently and the nervous system returns to its natural function.* Everything I'd learned about stress had taught me that the human nervous system has a tendency to get stuck in a low-grade state of flight-or-fight arousal that disturbs sleep, impairs digestion, inhibits organ function, and undermines well-being. When it comes to health, the primary purpose of pranayama is to free the ANS of this stress fixation and return it to a nimble state centered in rest-and-digest dominance.

Going one step further, the role of pranayama on the householder path came clear to me. Pranayama is a stage of yoga in which postures are coupled with breathwork to revitalize the nervous system and restore what SK called its *natural function.* The end of that stage is marked when a yogi can sit down, engage the breath, and reliably access the calm, clear mind that arises from a healthy ANS in a relaxed state of parasympathetic dominance. Yoga and Buddhism both call this state "equanimity" and describe it as "an evenness of mind." When equanimity is gained, the role of pranayama on a householder's path shifts. Some amount of breathwork will continue to be practiced alongside postures to keep the body healthy and the nervous system vital, balanced, and

[7] These slight variations are qualitatively different from the symptoms of heart arrythmia.

capable of self-regulation. But a householder's emphasis should shift to the subsequent stages of yoga focused on sitting meditation.[8]

APPLYING THIS IN PRACTICE

Several contemporary approaches to breathwork have grown popular and the principles underlying yogic pranayama can help inform all the different breath practices taught by today's teachers.[9] For a long time, I did pranayama dutifully because it was recognized as an important step on the path of yoga. All these years later, it's easy to list the reasons I continue to practice its classic techniques:

- Helps maintain the health, vigor, and vital capacity of my respiratory system in the face of aging.
- Preserves my energetic vitality by keeping my metabolism high and nervous system centered in a mild state of rest-and-digest dominance supportive of health.
- Keeps me breath-aware in daily life and less apt to trigger fight-or-flight in response to perceived threats.
- In times of challenge, enables me to generate the energy and focus required to act dynamically by slightly emphasizing my inhalations to activate the sympathetic nervous system.
- In times of overwhelm, gives me tools to quell mental agitation and promote physical relaxation and healing by emphasizing my exhalations to stimulate the parasympathetic nervous system.
- Enables me to smoothly enter meditation and experience moments of inner stillness when the breath grows faint, recedes into the background, and naturally falls out of awareness.

[8] As previously explained, the renunciate path is different. Pranayama will continue to be practiced intensively as its own form of dynamic meditation.

[9] Among the most popular practices are the physiological sigh, coherent breathing, sudharshana kriya as taught by the Art of Living Foundation, Tibetan tummo (fire breathing) and most notably the version of tummo taught by Wim Hof, box breathing, 4-7-8 breathing as taught by Dr. Andrew Weil, and humming bee breath.

The seed of a tree contains the organic pattern from which all its required roots, trunk, branches, leaves, flowers, and fruits will naturally take shape. In a similar way, the seed of the tree of yoga is pranayama. Instilled in its practice is the energetic pattern from which all the stages of meditation leading to samadhi will surely unfold.

APPENDIX 4

THE SHAT KRIYAS

The *shat kriyas* or *six purifying actions* are a comprehensive set of yogic cleansing techniques that graphically demonstrate the intensity with which the Indian sages pursued their ideal of internal hygiene. Versions of them are used in Ayurvedic medicine to improve bodily health, but in yoga their purpose was to prepare a student to practice anuloma viloma and other forms of pranayama. Before initiating a student into anuloma viloma, a traditional guru would assess their physical condition. Lean and highly-fit students would immediately be taught the technique and begin its practice. Less fit aspirants would be guided through the shat kriyas, each of which was intended to "churn" an area of the body to eliminate its buildup of toxic wastes.[1] Along with dulling vitality, the yogis believed these accumulated wastes, if substantial, could impede the practice of pranayama or even render it ineffective.

Through the practice of pranayama alone, all impurities will cease to exist. But yogic aspirants with an excess of fat, phlegm, mucous, bile, or other form of congestion face an obstacle. It is not easy for them to perform the purifying action of anuloma viloma successfully. It is for these aspirants that the six cleansing practices are taught. Neti, dhauti, basti, nauli, kapalabhati, tratak—these scientific techniques of cleansing the interior of the body were not derived through logic. They are the priceless discoveries of past sages who conducted yogic experiments. If learned directly from an able teacher, these practices will prove beneficial and aid well-being.

[1] While an established element of the yogic path, the role of the shat kriyas was not universally praised. Some teachers opposed their practice and favored an exclusive reliance on the purifying power of pranayama. For more on this point, see Hatha Yoga Pradipika verse 2.37. Some yoga schools call these the "shat karmas" or "six actions." The Sanskrit word *chalana* means churning.

Trying to do them from books is ill-advised and will surely do more harm than good. The bodily purification brought about by the correct practice of these yogic techniques is of a very high quality. It can clear up chronic diseases and even forge extraordinary qualities. Aspirants who need the help of the shat kriyas should seek out expert instruction from a yoga school, and then practice them correctly in solitude to prepare themselves for pranayama practice. Aspirants free of these excesses can become travelers on the path of pranayama straightaway.[2]

Neti is a word that in the context of the shat kriyas means *no toxins.* Neti practice cleanses the nasal passages and sinus cavities. The most popular version uses a neti pot to direct a flow of warm salt water into one nostril and out the other. A more invasive version uses a wax-coated string that is pushed into the nose and drawn out the mouth. Eleven different forms of *dhauti* (washing) cleanse the entire length of the alimentary canal including the mouth, teeth, tongue, food pipe, stomach, intestines, and rectum.[3] Centuries before toothbrushing became prevalent in the West, the yogis used soft twigs to carefully clean their teeth after meals. The best-known phase of dhauti involves swallowing then disgorging a sterilized cloth that is three inches wide and twenty feet long to soak up impurities from the stomach. *Basti* (lower region) cleanses the large intestine, colon, and anus through a water-method similar to enema. *Nauli* (rolling like a wave) invigorates the vital organs through a rigorous churning of the abdominal muscles. *Kapalabhati*

[2] Mucus as the word is commonly used comes from the upper airways, where phlegm comes from the lower airways. Phlegm is coughed up from the lungs and mucus is blown out of the nose. Bile is a bitter alkaline fluid that aids digestion and is secreted by the liver and stored in the gallbladder. The early yogis lacked this degree of physiological knowledge. They used the words *sleshma* to describe any of the thick liquid-like substances found in diseased bodies; *kaphadyarga*, a pathological expression of what they imagined to be a cementing substance that held the bones and joints together; and *karma* in the belief that a subtle residue or taint lodges in the body as a result of evil actions. All of these were seen to dull bodily aliveness and diminish mental awareness.

[3] As modern people, we can understand why the shat kriyas might be done to cleanse the physical body. But the yogis who developed them were equally interested in opening up the subtle body and especially its blocked central channel. When done in sequence, these practices generate intense feelings in all the chakra regions from anus to crown, and the increased physical sensitivity remaining afterward was seen to reflect a revitalization of the subtle body.

(skull-shining) is a breathing exercise said to stoke the inner fire and burn away impurities, which translates as increasing the rate of metabolism. If done vigorously, it clears the nostrils and stimulates the sinus cavities, and coupled with bhastrika pranayama was said to purify the brow chakra that we associate with the frontal lobes of the brain. *Tratak* (steady gazing) is practiced until tears form to cleanse the eyes, which was thought to enhance vision. In some yoga schools, tratak practice resumes in the early stages of yogic meditation, where the same technique is used to fixate attention on an external object and steady the mind.

It's noteworthy that even in the prime of his youth Swami Kripalu was not considered a lean and highly-fit aspirant. Instead of guiding him in the shat kriyas, his guru led SK through a six-month period of progressively restricted eating that ended with a 41-day water fast. Only after his successful completion of this lengthy fast was he initiated into the practice of anuloma viloma. Despite this personal history, it was clear from Swami Kripalu's talks and writings that he was familiar with all six of these techniques.[4]

Cloth-cleansing is a preliminary kriya done willfully before pranayama begins. Once I happened to be in Hardwar when a Bengali brother got in trouble. He had swallowed the cloth, but when trying to bring it out the cloth stopped coming and would not budge. He became afraid and started crying loudly. As he pulled, his throat resisted. In the tug of war, the blood started oozing. He was taken to a medical doctor who said, "This is a yogic kriya. I don't know how to help you." The doctor knew of me and while leading the man to where I was staying a crowd of people formed.

I had just come out of my meditation room when the doctor approached and told me what had happened. The brother could not talk, so he just held my feet. I said to him, "It is very simple. Just

[4] For more on SK's water fast and anuloma viloma initiation, see *Dharma Then Moksha*, Chapter 1. By far the best treatment of the shat kriyas I've encountered appears in a richly-illustrated book by Swami Kripalu's direct disciple, Swami Rajarshi Muni, titled *Classical Hatha Yoga*. The great majority of yoga teachers receive no training in the shat kriyas. Readers wanting to explore them in practice are advised to seek out an Ayurvedic center whose services are overseen by a traditionally trained Ayurvedic doctor.

follow my instructions. Take some water and swallow a little of the cloth back down." He refused out of fear that only more would go in, so I put my hand on his head to calm him and waited. For a long time, he wouldn't do it. But eventually he sipped some water and swallowed a little more. His clenched throat had formed the cloth into a ball. Once moistened by the water, the ball separated and within a short time the cloth came out. Before the crowd disbursed, another swami stood up from the crowd and loudly said, "Don't anybody dare do this." Swallowing the cloth is not inherently dangerous. If learned from an experienced teacher, it is promotive of health. But if you don't have a guru and learn from books, this kind of thing can happen.

The lifestyle of ashram residents included a number of purification techniques drawn from the shat kriyas. The foundational practice was a healthy diet with directions to fast, or eat a simple mono-diet of fruit or rice, one day per week. For many years, this discipline was supported by the kitchen, which prepared only simple and bland foods on Thursdays. When guest attendance rose in the late 1980s, a full menu had to always be available on the serving line. While weekly fasting remained an ashram ideal, it largely fell by the wayside in practice.[5]

If you really want to purify the body and attain to excellent health, refrain from eating one day of the week. It is best if you can take water and nothing else. If you can't do that, limit yourself to fruit juice, or milk, or replace your meals with a bowl of vegetable soup, or take moderate quantities of any one type of healthy food. If that is too difficult, just eat one healthy meal at mid-day, or stop eating junk foods entirely. One who learns to eat with discrimination and aspires to moderation in diet (mitahar) will take naturally to the practice of yoga and pranayama.

Most residents used a tongue cleaner each morning to scrape away the furry buildup deposited on the back of tongue during the night,

[5] John Mundahl is an early ashram resident who did this practice of weekly fasting. He wrote a guide based on Swami Kripalu's teachings called *Mastering the One-Day Fast: The Key to Health and Longevity.*

which is a form of *dhauti*. Many also used a neti pot to cleanse and keep the sinus passages open. The Kripalu Shop did a brisk business in selling these items, which back then were exotic but have since become commonplace. In Pennsylvania, the ashram's Health Center featured colonics to support the purification process brought on by a vegetarian diet, weekly fasting, and yoga practice. After moving to Massachusetts, the revamped Healing Arts Department ceased colonics to focus on massage. But the new facility included a men and women's sauna to purify the skin through sweating, both of which were always in use.

Fasting is a tool to remedy the overeating habit. If a person can truly practice moderation in diet, there is no need of fasting. I followed the same fasting practice that I ask of my students for many years. This was necessary because disciples were always bringing me different kinds of food. Even if I just ate one bite of everything, it still got to be too much. Without the respite of those fast days, I would have gotten sick. Prolonged fasting purifies the body, but it also weakens it. And when you start eating, the spring that you have stretched one way is likely to snap back, making you food-crazy and apt to resume eating in ways that keep the body impure. Now I am old and have accepted that a yogi has to practice moderation all the way to moksha (liberation). I take one meal a day and eat it carefully. I have made arrangements that no food is kept in my residence. I still need that kind of external support because the wisdom born of self-discipline only lasts so long. I am giving you this description of my eating habits at this late stage in my life only to clarify the subject of fasting and moderation in diet further.

Morning yoga at the ashram always included the duo of *uddiyana bandha* or "the flying up lock" and *agnisara dhauti*, often translated as "stomach pumping." In this kriya, the breath is expelled and held out, while the navel is repeatedly pulled back toward the spinal cord to stimulate the vital organs and kindle the digestive fire. This is a preparatory practice for *nauli* or abdominal churning, one of the most highly-praised shat kriyas. Morning meditation was preceded by two rounds of kapalabhati breathing, which led directly into a twelve-minute period of anuloma viloma, to prepare for a twelve-minute period of silent sitting.

While the full complement of shat kriyas was not available in the ashram, the emphasis on purification through healthy lifestyle and regular yoga practice was strong.

The sadhana done by SK in the secluded second half of his life aroused the primal energies of his body to a degree that led to the spontaneous practice of kriyas. These next-level kriyas are categorically different from the volitional six cleansing action, and he graphically explains how.

The continual practice of pranayama eventually stirs the kundalini power into activity generating spontaneous kriyas that are natural and more effective than the shat kriyas. For example, in the early days of my practice I experienced rubbing kriya, in which the root of the tongue is rubbed with the index finger. This makes the dregs of phlegm and bile come up from the stomach of their own accord to be expelled by means of the mouth. Even doing cloth-cleansing several times cannot remove as many impurities as are expelled in one effort through the rubbing method. This is an example of why many sages give greater importance to performing pranayama than to the six practices.

It is incorrect to think of these kriyas as an early and transient phase of renunciate yoga. One of the chief kriyas mentioned by Swami Kripalu is *anahat nada* (unstruck sound), which is the chanting of unscripted sounds, melodies, and mantras. In various talks delivered in America, he describes this kriya occurring late in his life and after thirty years of intensive practice.

I apologize for my singing this morning. For many days, different yogic kriyas have been happening in meditation, and sometimes they affect my throat. Neither do I select the words, or the tune, or desire even to sing. This is pure sound born from within. It can be said these yogic kriyas happen spontaneously, but only after many willful actions have been taken by an aspirant to purify their mind and body. One's consciousness is naturally drawn to some particular region of the body. Then the prana (life force) goes there to produce the kriya, which further purifies the subtle body. The results of a kriya may go unrecognized as it is taking place, but eventually they become evident. Although these kriyas happen through the medium of prana, they have their origin in the spiritual source from which the body receives its energy. The end stage of purification is a yogi's wholehearted surrender to that divine source (Ishvara pranidhana).

These spontaneous cleansing actions suggest the willfully-done shat kriyas may have originated as attempts to mirror and replicate the nature-born experiences of gifted yogis like SK.

APPENDIX 5

A BRIEF HISTORY OF THE TERM SAMADHI

The roots of yoga predate written history and very little is known about its origins. The first references to yoga-like themes appear in the Vedas, which were orally passed down for generations before being composed in Sanskrit around 1500 BCE. The Vedas are a cryptic collection of ritualistic hymns and sacrificial utterances whose meaning has largely been lost. The first written sources relevant to today's yoga practitioners are the Upanishads, which were composed over several centuries starting as early as 800 BCE. The word *Upanishad* means "to sit at the feet of a master" and this remarkable collection of over one hundred texts preserve the dialogues between sages living as forest hermits and their disciples.

Samadhi is explained in the earliest Upanishads by distinguishing it from the three universally-known states of consciousness: waking, dreaming, and deep dreamless sleep. In these teachings, samadhi is referred to as *turiya*, which literally means "the fourth." But this should not be taken to mean that samadhi is a fourth and independent state on par with the others. Turiya exposes a yogi to the primordial and unconditioned consciousness that is the substratum of the other three. Turiya initially presents as an illuminating but transient meditative state. As such, it does not reflect a lasting realization. Later Upanishads describe its culmination in *turiya titha*, which means "that which is beyond the fourth," to reflect its full expression as a stable trait.[1] This corresponds to

[1] Turiya is discussed in the Chandogya, Mandukya, Brihadaranyaka, and Maitri Upanishads. The fifteenth-century Hatha Yoga Pradipika attempts to integrate yoga's past teachings into a coherent approach. Verse 4.3-4 lists turiya as one of samadhi's many synonyms.

the teachings of Swami Kripalu, who recognizes two similar categories of samadhi.

A close student once asked me a good question, "What is the difference between sleep and samadhi?" Yoga recognizes four primary states of consciousness. In the waking state, a multitude of thought waves move through the mind stemming from our sense perceptions. In the dream state, a smaller number of thought waves move through the mind drawn from our memory bank of sensory impressions. In deep dreamless sleep, the flow of thoughts stops so the mind can rest undisturbed. Only upon waking do you recall it as being blissful. Samadhi is called "the fourth state." Like deep sleep, it is thoughtless, but samadhi is also entirely different, because in it you remain fully conscious. While this explanation may expand your understanding, you have to enter samadhi to really recognize the difference. In deep sleep, a person comes back to the waking state feeling well-rested, with all their faculties as they were before. But after samadhi, a yogi returns to the waking state with higher wisdom and will cease performing actions in life that are motivated by ignorance.

Buddhism arose in the middle of the Upanishadic era and uses the word *samadhi* to describe a state of highly-focused or one-pointed concentration. While its three main schools of Theravadin, Mahayana, and Vajrayana Buddhism vary considerably, most adherents accept the earliest Theravadin teachings in which samadhi is cultivated through a consistent practice of awareness-focusing meditation in which the *Four Foundations of Mindfulness* are contemplated. These are mindfulness of the body; mindfulness of feelings; mindfulness of mind states; and mindfulness of the Four Noble Truths taught in the discourses of the historical Buddha, which are collectively called *The Dharma*.[2]

The Mahayana school of Zen Buddhism includes a curious description of the movement into realization as "a backward step." This closely

[2] According to tradition, the Buddha lived from 563-483 BCE. Scholars suggest he may have lived as much as a century later. After renouncing the world, the prince Siddhartha Gautama became an ascetic and studied with various yoga masters prior to attaining nirvana. While his dharma is widely recognized as a new and revolutionary revelation, Buddha can rightly be called a yogi. Along with samadhi, his teachings include many elements drawn from the older Vedic and yoga traditions.

parallels the idea that our hidden potential for samadhi dwells in the immediacy prior to all experience. Like yoga, Zen recognizes two stages of samadhi. The first is *kensho*, a descriptive Japanese word that means "a flash of lightning on a dark night that makes the landscape visible" and points to a sudden but ephemeral illumination. The second is *satori*, which means "awakening" and refers to a steady state of realization.

The approach to cultivating samadhi adopted by the Vajrayana school of Tibetan Buddhism could be described as all-encompassing. It includes energy awakening and raising elements drawn from Shaivite kundalini yoga, sitting meditation techniques that cultivate both cognitive insight and empathic compassion, and innovative rituals of deity worship performed through intricate visualizations. While samadhi plays a pivotal role in all forms of Buddhism, it is not considered the end state. Samadhi is the meditative means to realize the emptiness of all phenomena and gain nirvana through blowing out the fire of greed, hatred, and delusion said to lie at the root of the egocentric self.

In India, the noble Lord Buddha is called "the wise one." After renouncing the world, he did a very deep sadhana. Attaining nirvana, he extinguished the discontent of the mind-based self and discovered these guiding principles: suffering exists; suffering has a cause; and suffering can be removed. Then he taught this dharma that brings an end to suffering all over India. Later his influence spread to China, Japan, Tibet, and many other countries. All over the world, Lord Buddha is renowned as a sage who used meditation to perfect his concentration and obtain liberating knowledge in samadhi.

Despite its antiquity, yoga was only accepted as a one of India's six classical philosophies (shad darshana) through the work of the brilliant sage Patanjali, who is credited with authoring the Yoga Sutra, which scholars date to 200 CE. In codifying the yogic approach, Patanjali drew heavily on *Sankhya*, a dualistic system of thought that distinguishes between two fundamental categories of existence: *purusha* and *prakriti*.[3]

[3] A text called the Sankhya Karika is said to have been written by sage Kapila in the Upanishadic era. Patanjali drew from this and other pre-existing sources, many of which have been lost. Even the eight-limbs (ashtangha) of his yogic path are not original, as they appear in earlier Upanishads. Patanjali's classical yoga is qualitatively different from Ashtanga Vinyasa, the popular form of asana-based hatha yoga devel-

Purusha is the pure consciousness of spirit. Prakriti is the primordial matter from which material creation unfolds in an orderly set of downward steps. As prakriti descends into material form, three *gunas (strands)* emerge that are inherently unstable. Sankhya describes the three gunas as the constantly-shifting substrate of all matter, much like the subatomic trio of neutron-proton-electron recognized by contemporary science. Mistakenly identifying with the ever-changing body and mind (prakriti), we are certain to suffer. But in truth we are neither body nor mind, we are the immaterial and changeless spirit (purusha).

Sankhya has been accepted as an integral part of yoga philosophy that views the entire universe as born from two primary elements. Purusha is the eternal and unchanging source. Prakriti is nature, which is constantly in flux because of the activity of the three gunas. When attraction or aversion arises in the mind of a Sankhya yogi, he believes with a strong conviction, "I am the inactive and liberated Purusha. The actions of this body and mind are not my actions, they are owned by nature. I am merely the witness of these actions." By overcoming mental disturbances in this way, the Sankhya yogi activates discriminative intelligence (buddhi) and attains steadiness of mind (samadhi). Without such steadiness, Self-realization and liberation are impossible.

Where Sankhya explains how a soul descends into form, Patanjali presents the reverse process through which a soul can ascend the metaphysical ladder of creation to free itself from material entanglement. His school of Classical Yoga is a path of meditation in which seated asanas and pranayama are used to steady the mind. Through intensive concentration, all mental activities, and the fluctuations in consciousness they produce, are gradually attenuated. Samadhi results from ardent meditation practice (abhyasa) performed with an attitude of mental detachment (vairagya). In with-seed samadhi, these fluctuations are temporarily suppressed. In without-seed samadhi, the subconscious activators (samskaras) believed to cause these mental fluctuations are uprooted, bringing them forever to an end.

---

oped by K. Pattabhi Jois (1915-2009).

It's important to note that in Classical Yoga the outcome of samadhi is not any kind of merger or union. Instead, it's the complete separation of the individual soul from its involvement with the constantly-changing and thus illusory material world born of the gunas. Samadhi is the means to the end state of *kaivalya,* the ecstatic aloneness of the purusha freed from its ignorance and material bondage. While Sankhya philosophy is non-theistic, Patanjali recognizes that samadhi and kaivalya can also occur through *Ishvara pranidhana*, which means "fixing attention on or surrendering to the Lord." This introduction of a supreme being into yoga was a bold attempt by Patanjali to reconcile the competing views prevalent in his time, which included dualism and nondualism, as well as theism and non-theism. The Yoga Sutra brings these systems together by emphasizing their many points of agreement. This gives yoga practitioners latitude to choose a guiding philosophical orientation and tailor their practice of meditative concentration accordingly.

Sage Patanjali teaches us in his aphorisms that withdrawing the mind from all external disturbances by focusing on an object of contemplation is the best means of attaining mental peace, and with that will come happiness. In his commentary, Maharishi Vyasa says this is a truth that everyone can practice. When our mind is outwardly engaged through the senses, it is easily disturbed. When our mind is detached from the senses by the techniques of yoga, it naturally grows still and peaceful. A yogi intent on samadhi concentrates their attention on an object of meditation until nothing but that exists in their consciousness. Doing this practice, their mind passes through many different states. After intense practice, a meditating yogi forgets even themself and becomes completely identified with their object of contemplation. This is known as samadhi, which Patanjali defines as the complete stoppage of the thought process. The peace of a yogi who knows how to enter samadhi and abide in the superconscious state is never disturbed.

Indian religion includes a stunning multiplicity of sects, but the dominant one by far is called *Vedanta.*[4] Vedanta literally means "the

[4] Vedanta is a living tradition that is still evolving today. Most schools accept the Bhagavad Gita as a divinely inspired text. It is part of the larger Mahabharat (Great

end of the Vedas," a name that aligns it with these time-honored texts. Vedanta is extolled for distilling the wisdom of the Vedas and Upanishads down to its essence. Orthodox Vedanta is a theistic approach that defines samadhi as the blissful merging of the individual soul or self (jivatma) with the macrocosmic oversoul and Supreme Self (Paramatman). In Vedantic yoga, samadhi is pursued through a coupling of devotional worship with daily meditation on one's chosen form of God. This form is called *ishta devata*, which literally means *one's cherished or preferred deity*. Meditation is often supported by a mantra containing the name of the deity and a *murti* or sacred image, both of which are used as objects of contemplation. Samadhi is initially experienced as a rapturous state of divine communion. If ardently pursued, it will lead to a second samadhi in which the formless Brahman is realized and a liberating absolute truth is revealed.

Yogi Yajnavalkya defines samadhi as the union of the individual soul with God. This is completely correct, but it must be technically understood. A person practicing devotional yoga enters with-seed (sabija) samadhi and experiences God with-form (saguna Brahman). This manifestation of God arises in the mind and is characterized by many virtuous and beneficent qualities. In India, there are many saints who attain to this blissful level and feel they have reached the highest, but this is not the final step. Only in without-seed (nirbija) samadhi is the God who is without attributes (nirguna Brahman) known. Only in this no-mind samadhi do the Supreme Self and individual consciousness really become one. There is nothing beyond that.

Vedanta gained prominence during the time of the Upanishads, but its influence waned with the growing popularity of Buddhism. In the eighth century, a monk named Shankara traversed the Indian subcontinent reviving the Vedic wisdom through his discourses and public debates. Historians credit Shankara with consolidating the ideas found

---

India) epic that scholars believe was composed between 200 BCE and 200 CE. Verse 2.54 of the Gita uses the term *samadhi-sthasya* to describe one who is steady in thought and steadfast in meditation. The sixth chapter provides practical instruction in meditation. In the Gita, samadhi is seen as the meditative means to achieve the ultimate goals of Vedantic yoga: Self-realization and God-realization.

in the Upanishads into a distinctive approach to Self-realization known as Advaita Vedanta. The word *advaita* means *not two* and it is often called "the path of non-duality." Meditation proceeds along a path of exclusion and dis-identification from the body and mind referred to as *neti neti* (not this, not this). While Advaita has its own approach to yoga and is based on a distinctive set of teachings, it remains part of Vedanta.

Swami Vivekananda introduced Advaita Vedanta to the West in his famous 1894 address to the world parliament of religions. Ever since it has grown and flourished as one of the most popular forms of Western yoga. In today's yoga world, there are also teachers of *neo-Advaita* who depart from its established teaching methodologies to speak directly from their own realization. Where traditional Advaita required twelve years of preliminary study and yoga practice before its deeper non-dual teachings would be transmitted to a student, neo-Vedanta is generally taught to anyone with sufficient interest to read a book or attend a workshop. Neo-Advaita is often criticized for encouraging students to mistake an initial and intellectual awakening for a true realization, which requires access to levels of awareness that Swami Kripalu described as *beyond-mind.*

Everyone must start upon the path of yoga from the experience of duality. If I as a teacher were to tell you as a student that all of existence is not-two, there is someone telling who thinks he knows and someone listening who is supposed to believe. This is not advaita. Yet there is a path to realize that we are not the body, nor our actions, nor our thoughts, and not even the observer (drsta) of our thoughts. Walking this path is a little like a passenger on a train who decides to find out who is driving. First, the passenger must make his way through all the intervening train cars to the locomotive. Finally entering the locomotive, the passenger goes to the front compartment and finds the engineer standing off to the side with his head out the window. In that moment, it doesn't seem that anyone is driving the train. Do not fool yourself into witnessing your thoughts and believing that you are the non-dual Brahman. Even in samadhi, the sense of 'I' exists until the very end. As long as the "I" exists, there will also be "others" and "the world." Understand that a subtle duality will prevail until the end of with-seed samadhi. Only in without-seed samadhi does the mind become no-mind and the mind-based self merge into the true Self. As a result, duality disappears and the non-dual state arises. But remember that in advaita there is no observer at all, so don't expect to be there to see it.

A new philosophy called Tantra arose around 500 CE to offer a fresh perspective on the relationship of ultimate truth and the material world in which we live. Tantra is founded on the view that worldly life does not have to be renounced in favor of spiritual awakening. Tantra's life-affirming stance was a marked departure from earlier yogic philosophies. Sankhya views the human soul as trapped in matter. Vedanta sees the world of the senses as a dangerous and beguiling illusion. In many systems like these, spirituality can only be sought by a person willing to renounce the world and its pleasures. Instead of asceticism, Tantra celebrates embodiment and approves of enjoyment, avoiding the inner splits, inhibitions, and complexes that self-denial often creates.

The founders of Tantra conceptualized consciousness and matter as two poles on a cosmic continuum. They symbolized these poles as *Shiva*, the masculine principle of consciousness, and *Shakti,* the feminine principle of creative energy. Within the microcosm of the individual, Shiva is the pure awareness that underlies the ego, and Shakti is the life force that sustains the body and vivifies its subtle energy centers and health-sustaining functions. Tantra depicts Shiva and Shakti as cosmic lovers, drawn together by their opposite qualities. The splendor of the macrocosmic universe is the outpouring of their ecstatic lovemaking. Seeing spirit and matter as connected by a unifying love is what enabled the founders of Tantra to pioneer a life-affirming philosophy that trusts human life will naturally lead to spiritual awakening if lived joyously and savored.

Back to the time of the Vedas, Indians practiced religious rituals that combined meditative awareness with the use of *mandalas (*circles creating sacred space), *mantras* (sacred words and sounds), *mudras* (expressive gestures), and the worship of various gods and goddesses. The teachers of Tantra created a new repertoire of rituals designed to transform the consciousness of their students. Many of these rituals were unorthodox and especially potent because they ran counter to prevailing religious norms. Practicing them, students would confront powerful emotions such as terror, shock, lust, and awe that swiftly carried them into beyond-mind meditation. After Tantric meditation is ritually initiated, it proceeds along a path of inclusion referred to as *asmi asmi* (*this too, this too*). On this path the body-mind is embraced as a manifestation of the divine, dispelling the myth of separateness that divides reality into artificial distinctions like matter and spirit.

The practice of yoga is the trunk of the tree of Indian spirituality. All its religions including Buddhism and Jainism are but branches. Tantra began as a system of mystical rites in which the universal male and female principles were considered deities and their respective qualities worshipped. The roots of these rites are ancient and pre-date Buddhism. It is these rites that centuries later developed into Tantric Hatha Yoga, which spread all over India. Today the word yoga is associated with the Vedas and Upanishads, but the way yoga is practiced comes more from Tantra. In this approach, the life energy is considered feminine and called Shakti. When made steady and strong, Shakti energy begins to ascend the central channel in the spine. When it reaches the uppermost energy center in the head, Shakti meets her beloved Shiva. The action of inhaling and exhaling stops, and the yogi enters the first samadhi. In this samadhi, the mind begins to lose its power to distract and deceive by creating contrivance. Eventually, the yogi sees that there is no separation between the life-giving energy of Shakti and the consciousness of Shiva. This leads to the second samadhi, which in Tantra is called the arisen state (vyutthana avastha). Even though the body and breath move again, the yogi remains stable in the state of Divine union. While Tantra does not shun worldly enjoyment, a true tantric adept is not a licentious person but a realized being of perfect self-control.

Tantra produced a cultural renaissance but eventually fell into disrepute. Current research attributes this to the wrong action of scandalous teachers and a ritual system that grew overly complex and expensive. Despite its downfall, aspects of Tantra's philosophical innovations have been adopted by all the major yoga schools. Authentic Tantra is qualitatively different from the sexual practices often called neo-Tantra, which draw on various yoga-like techniques to increase sexual pleasure.

Hatha Yoga is an offshoot of Tantra that can be traced to sage Matsyendra and his successor, sage Goraksha, who lived around 1000 CE when the Tantric movement had grown stagnant. Matsyendra and Goraksha recast Tantra in yogic terms by developing three primary rituals: *asana* (postures and their full expression as mudras or energy seals), *pranayama* (breath regulation), and *dhyana* (meditation). A student could learn how to practice these rituals again and again to catalyze their spiritual growth. The Tantric word conveying this orientation to sustained practice is *sadhana*, which means "the systematic practice of spiritual disciplines for self-transformation."

Drawing on the work of earlier systems, the adepts of Hatha Yoga refined the model of the subtle body that is now universally embraced by yoga. The goal of their yoga was to raise the primal energy from root to crown, piercing each energy center and causing it to blossom into vivid aliveness. When the primal energy reaches the head, it dissolves all the rigid structures of the mind. Shakti merges with Shiva, and the yogi experiences *samadhi* (Divine union). SK often spoke about his own practice of samadhi in these terms and described how the bridge of the dualistic witness could be quickly crossed when meditation was supercharged by the movement of energy into the highest centers of consciousness.

Through continually performing the yogic rites of hatha yoga, the life energy is made to flow in the central channel. When this flow starts to fly upward, it is the harbinger of victory. Sage Svatmarama describes it as a powerful bird that begins to tirelessly soar up. As the life energy becomes established in the brain, the movement of breath grows faint and meditative absorption begins. When the flow of breath ceases, a practitioner reaches the limit of with-seed samadhi. The perception of God continues as energy coalesces at the ajna chakra, where you, God, and the universe are still separate. As soon as the energy (Shakti) reaches the thousand-petal chakra, it merges with consciousness (Shiva) and there is only God alone. This is true advaita (non-duality). With no one left to observe it, this cannot rightly be called an experience. A practitioner who stays continually in this God-alone state is liberated within six months.

Hatha Yoga flourished for a few centuries before gradually fading. Its teachings are best preserved in the *Hatha Yoga Pradipika,* a text written in the Middle Ages that scholars believe is a compilation of earlier sources lost to history. Several of its verses can be read to praise a state of samadhi in which the body becomes rigid, the breath ceases, and the mind is rendered thoughtless. SK cautioned against this interpretation of samadhi:

Here it is appropriate to mention what is called jada samadhi, a kind of swoon in which the body remains still and the mind becomes unconscious. This state is sometimes encountered by a yogi who keeps his body straight and stiff, often by willfully concentrating attention between the eyebrows. If a yogi mistakes this thoughtless state for the genuine samadhi, they may go on practicing it for a long time. Some yogis learn to remain continuously that way. Like a person in a coma, they do not feel hunger or thirst. Moreover, the breathing process may stop, enabling the yogi to remain buried under the ground for a few days or even a few months. Accomplishing feats like this may lead a yogi to claim that he has achieved the highest samadhi, but this is delusion. It is true that the body of a yogi in samadhi does not move, and their mind remains in a thoughtless state. But these are superficial similarities. The true measure of samadhi is the level of consciousness attained by the yogi. A yogi entering swoons becomes unconscious, while a yogi entering samadhi becomes superconscious. Only the latter yogi will receive the highest wisdom (ritambhara prajna) that grants them Self-realization (atman vijnana) and liberation (moksha).

APPENDIX 6

DIVINE DESCENT AND ASCENT MEDITATION

This potent protocol for reliably accessing depth meditation comes from the Himalayan sages. It is based on the view that meditation is a tool to embody the sacred energy of spirit. According to these sages, this spiritual energy enters our manifest being through various brain centers and only comes into conscious awareness when the nerve centers and neural pathways of the body open to allow its free flow through the chakra system which can be seen as the central and autonomic nervous systems. The process is similar to turning on a series of light switches that enable electrical current to move through a network of wires and circuitry.

Although reading this technique may make it seem cumbersome or complex, it is a simple process of first scanning the body from top to bottom, and then directing the attention to rise from bottom to top. Starting out, it can be helpful to begin the descent by imagining that someone poured warm honey on the top of your head and you are tracking its slow downward flow through the force of gravity. Similarly, the ascent can be thought of as a gradual process of filling the interior of the body with vital breath-based energy. Once you are familiar with the process, it becomes easy to remember and feels quite natural.

1. Take Your Seat: Adjust your sitting position to make the body comfortable. Press the sitting bones down, slightly tuck the chin, and lift through the crown of your head to elongate the spine. Close the eyes to facilitate inner focus.

2. Move into Belly Breathing: Take a minute to simply notice how you are already breathing. Then locate the spot in the torso where you feel the flow of breath most acutely. Watching the breath move in and out, invite this spot to gradually soften, facilitating an easy movement of the belly and diaphragm. As you continue to watch the breath, you'll find your body naturally moving into a body-based breath that does not require any mental monitoring. Once this breath pattern establishes itself, you are ready to engage this or any meditation technique.

3. Divine Descent: Raise your inner awareness to the area of the head above the eyebrows. Notice the spaciousness and inner silence that comes from focusing your awareness in this way. Rest for a few moments in this state. When the mind begins to wander, invite this beyond-mind energy and awareness to descend by flowing into and energizing the following body parts:

Eyes	Wrists	Diaphragm
Temples	Hands and fingers	Belly
Ears	Forearms	Pelvis
Nose	Upper Arms	Hips
Lips and Mouth	Shoulders	Thighs
Jaw	Tip of Tongue	Calves and Shins
Top of Shoulders	Throat	Feet
Elbows	Chest	Toes

When you reach the toes, allow the energy and awareness to complete its descent to the very core and center of your body-mind, however you experience that bedrock level of your being.

4. Divine Ascent: Now allow the energy and awareness to steadily ascend as you consciously relax and let go of any control over the following body parts and nerve centers:

Toes	Navel Center	Shoulders
Ankles	Fingers and Hands	Heart Center
Knees	Wrists	Throat Center
Hips	Forearms	Soft Palate
Root Center	Elbows	Third Eye Center
Sex Center	Upper Arms	Crown Center

5. Rest in the Beyond-Mind State: As possible, set aside any mental activity and rest in the spaciousness of the beyond-mind state. Tremendous power and intelligence can flow into us in moments of stillness and silence. Depth meditation is an unforced and spontaneous happening. You have done the best anyone can do, which is to establish the conditions for it to occur. Learn to release the habit of focusing on whatever sensations, thoughts, or feelings are passing through the foreground of the mind. Step back into the background consciousness that underlies and surrounds the thinking mind. This is called "meditation without support." It is an advanced practice that only comes from non-doing.

6. The Still Point and the Non-Dual Field: When illumined by meditative awareness, the still point of personal awareness can expand into the vast field-of-all-possibility that is sometimes called the non-dual field. The wave disappears into the ocean; the soul becomes one with God; the individual Atman realizes its unity with the cosmic Brahman; the world's wisdom traditions overflow with similar descriptions. This is a mysterious process that spans a spectrum of simple intimacy with self to rapturous states of communion and union. Give up any striving to get somewhere and let the truth be revealed in your own direct experience of being.

7. Skillful Use of Bodily Anchor, Breath Awareness, Mantra and Inquiry: The nondual field is paradoxical. It is absolutely still and unchanging, yet it also has unpatterned fluctuations that cause life force to move, breath to flow, and sensations, thoughts, and feelings to arise and pass through the mind. In order to rest in the field of all possibility, you will need to learn to practice "meditation with support" through the skillful use of subtle tools such as bodily anchor, breath awareness, mantra, and inquiry. For example, you might lightly anchor your awareness at a physical spot such as the heart center. Simply register anything that naturally arises in the compassion of the heart space and let it go. If thoughts distract, you can mentally repeat a word such as "peace" one time to disrupt their flow and return to spacious awareness. If thoughts persist, as they often do, you can repeat the word in a rhythm with the breath. If your awareness drifts, you can use the tool of inquiry by asking yourself a question such as, "What is true here?" A good question not only sharpens your awareness but directs it toward a more profound connection to reality. The practice is to remain absorbed in beyond-mind meditation as much as possible until the end of session. Find your own ways to do this.

8. Come Out of Meditation Gently: Gradually deepen the breath. Take a few moments to register, reflect upon, and integrate your experience. Stretch in a way that feels good to establish yourself in your normal, embodied awareness before moving on to whatever is next for you.

***

If you draw a straight line connecting the eyebrows, the area of the head above this line can be called the Absolute space or the realm of God. This is the domain of depth meditation.

***

In yoga books both ancient and modern, there are descriptions of various energy centers. It is by activating these centers that the science of meditation is produced. When all the energy centers are active, a ladder is formed. Whatever type of meditation you practice, your ascent of this ladder must begin with the lowest energy center. One who fully activates the highest center ascends to the complete end of the path; there is nothing beyond that.

***

Depth meditation leads to nirodha, a cutting-off of all input from the mind and senses. The yogi enters a state beyond time and space, a state beyond waking and dreaming, a state of pure knowledge. Such a yogi is said to have gone above death and knows from his own direct experience that what we perceive as time and space, movement and stillness, observer and observed, desire and aversion, are all aspects of an undivided Absolute.

– Swami Kripalu

Richard Faulds, MA, JD, has practiced yoga and meditation for forty-five years in close association with Kripalu Center for Yoga & Health in Massachusetts. He has served as Kripalu's president, CEO, board chair, in house legal counsel, and a senior faculty member. Richard is also the author of *Kripalu Yoga: A Guide to Practice On and Off the Mat* and numerous other books on the Kripalu tradition including *Swami Kripalu's Yoga of Success and Self-Realization* published by Monkfish in 2025.

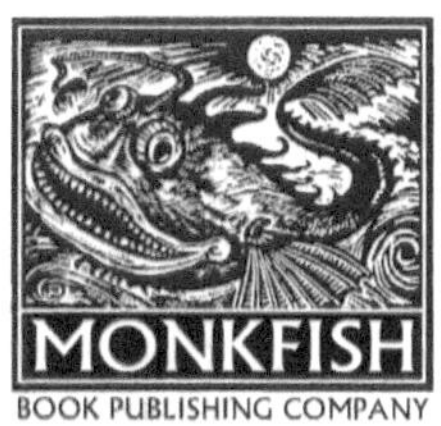

We are

Monkfish Book Publishing

...an independent press publishing spiritual and literary books from a diverse range of perspectives. Genres include memoirs, wisdom literature, fiction, and scholarly works of thought. Monkfish books appeal to the seasoned or novice seeker as well as to the general public looking for reliable sources on spirituality. The readers we had in mind when we began Monkfish in 2002 were devoted spiritual seekers, the type whose passion for the spiritual quest would lead them to read across a dazzling array of traditions: Buddhist, Hindu, Jewish, Christian, Muslim, Native American and more. It has always been our intent to publish works of spiritual authenticity for the general public as well as the specialist and scholar.

Our books are available from booksellers everywhere.

Use this QR code to see recently published books:

Use this one to sign-up for our monthly newsletter:

www.ingramcontent.com/pod-product-compliance
Lightning Source LLC
LaVergne TN
LVHW050952080826
845145LV00005B/1476

* 9 7 8 1 9 6 6 6 0 8 1 3 4 *